A friend of mine went to the racetrack with her husband when she had been on my program exactly one week. Between the front entrance and her seat she passed stands selling hot dogs, pizza, ice cream, Oriental food, soft drinks, beer, and candy. She survived this onslaught by bringing her own fruit and munching on it whenever temptation threatened.

They spent the day in the restaurant overlooking the track. But sitting at a dining table with friends all day didn't overwhelm her. In fact, she joined right in. Her drinks were iced tea and diet soda, and she chose her food carefully. ("Why didn't I order that?" her friends asked, when they compared their deep-fried crab cakes and their greasy beef with her delicate poached salmon.) As the hours passed and they lingered around the table, she popped an occasional grape.

She had a delightful day and she came out ahead.
—*DAVID LIEDERMAN*

"Here at last is a sensible, satisfying plan for dining deliciously while losing weight."
—*Florence Fabricant, food critic*

"No one I know understands food like David Liederman. And with recipes like Roasted Mushrooms and Garlic, and Roast Chicken Chez Louis, we can be orgiastic and prudent at the same meal. What a happy combination."
—*Michael Tucker, actor and producer*

St. Martin's Paperbacks titles are available at quantity discounts for sales promotions, premiums or fund raising. Special books or book excerpts can also be created to fit specific needs.

For information write to special sales manager, St. Martin's Press, 175 Fifth Avenue, New York, N.Y. 10010.

David's® LOSE WEIGHT PERMANENTLY, REDUCE YOUR CHOLESTEROL, AND STILL EAT 97% OF THE FOOD YOU LOVE DIET

(published in hardcover as *David's® Delicious Weight-Loss Program*)

DAVID LIEDERMAN WITH JOAN SCHWARTZ

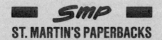

ST. MARTIN'S PAPERBACKS

NOTE: If you purchased this book without a cover you should be aware that this book is stolen property. It was reported as 'unsold and destroyed' to the publisher, and neither the author nor the publisher has received any payment for this 'stripped book'.

Before beginning this or any other medical or nutritional regimen, consult your physician to be sure it is appropriate for you.

The information in this book reflects the author's experiences and is not intended to replace medical advice. Any questions on symptoms, general or specific, should be addressed to your physician.

Fish Stock and Reduction and Chicken Stock and Reduction (Glace de poisson and Glace de volaille in the original recipes) reprinted from *Cooking the Nouvelle Cuisine in America*. Copyright © 1979 by Michèle Urvater and David Liederman. Reprinted by permission of Workman Publishing Company. All rights reserved.

This book was published in hardcover under the title *David's Delicious Weight-Loss Program*.

DAVID'S LOSE WEIGHT PERMANENTLY, REDUCE YOUR CHOLESTEROL, AND STILL EAT 97% OF THE FOOD YOU LOVE DIET

Copyright © 1990 by David Liederman and Joan Schwartz.

All rights reserved. No part of this book may be used or reproduced in any manner whatsoever without written permission except in the case of brief quotations embodied in critical articles or reviews. For information address St. Martin's Press, 175 Fifth Avenue, New York, N.Y. 10010.

Library of Congress Catalog Card Number: 89-77685

ISBN: 0-312-92573-5

Printed in the United States of America

St. Martin's Press hardcover edition published 1990
St. Martin's Paperbacks edition/August 1991

10 9 8 7 6 5 4 3 2 1

This book is dedicated to the tens of millions of people who have struggled with the eating compulsion and who are attempting to change their lives; and to our families, with love.

Contents

Acknowledgments — ix

Foreword — xi

PART ONE THE EATING SICKNESS

Chapter One
How This Program Can Help You — 3

Chapter Two
My Life as a Compulsive Eater — 10

Chapter Three
Up and Down on the Diet Seesaw — 32

PART TWO YOUR ROAD TO RECOVERY

Chapter Four
Trigger Foods: Name Your Poison — 47

Chapter Five
The Cholesterol Connection — 60

Chapter Six
David's Delicious Food Program ... 74

Chapter Seven
Get Moving ... 102

Chapter Eight
The New You: Guidelines and Strategies ... 116

Chapter Nine
Nothing But the Best: Eating Away from Home ... 132

• PART THREE   COOKING WITH DAVID •

Chapter Ten
Cooking with David ... 159

The Recipes	170
Stocks and Reductions	173
Soups	180
Salads	186
Pasta	193
Pizza	203
Fish and Shellfish	209
Poultry	221
Vegetables	233
Condiments	250
Fruit	253
Snacks and Fallbacks	258
Muffins and Cookies	261

Index ... 265

ACKNOWLEDGMENTS

We sincerely thank:
Dr. Charles Steinberg for being the catalyst for this project; Jane Dystel, our dynamo agent, for encouraging us and introducing us to Toni Lopopolo, our talented editor. Toni contributed her wit, wisdom, and patience to help shape this book. Susan Liederman, who helped create many of the delicious recipes and who provided insights into the biographical portions of the book.

Finally we thank each other for unstinting hard work and unflagging high spirits.

FOREWORD

As a practitioner of internal medicine and infectious disease in New York City for almost twenty years, I have dealt in my daily routine with a gamut of illness varying from the exotic to the mundane. In the current epidemic of Lyme disease in the Northeast and its attendant publicity, David Liederman's visit to my office with tick in hand proved to be mundane. What was exotic, however, was that before me stood over three hundred pounds of "cookie man" who, since his last visit to me some five years before, truly had come to exemplify the old saying, "You are what you eat."

After a physical exam and initial laboratory evaluation, it was apparent that David's obesity was accompanied by significantly high levels of cholesterol and blood sugar. I urged him to embark upon a strenuous diet and referred him to the Lipid Research Unit at New York Hospital-Cornell University Medical Center. Their evaluation confirmed David's hyperlipidemia and he was placed in the hands of a nutritionist. Several visits later, however, he informed me that he could do better himself—a phrase that inevitably brings forth a feeling of dismay from any physician dealing with an obese patient.

What evolved was not only a surprise, but also one of the most gratifying experiences one can have in the practice of medicine. David managed to lose over one hundred pounds. He did this with the realization that what was necessary was not just an avoidance of certain foods, but an entire modification of his eating habits.

David Liederman's philosophy is spelled out in a witty, easily readable, and informative narrative. He describes his ascendency to the realm of a three-hundred-pound fat man and identifies the importance of behavior patterns, trigger foods, cholesterol modification, and exercise in achieving and maintaining successful weight loss.

David's credo essentially provides a prescription for healthy living applicable to everyone, not just compulsive eaters. More important, it shows that change can be accomplished without giving up a lifetime of enjoyable eating.

—Charles Steinberg, M.D.
Associate Professor of Clinical Medicine, Cornell University Medical College; Associate Attending Physician, New York Hospital

■ PART ONE ■

THE EATING SICKNESS

Chapter One

How This Program Can Help You

A tick probably saved my life. During the last few years, the area around my country home in Westchester County, New York, has become overrun with deer. Ticks, some carrying dangerous Lyme disease, attach themselves to the deer and get an exciting ride through the woods. If you walk in the woods or even in the tall grass, the ticks may attach themselves to you.

One December morning my wife, Susan, noticed a very small tick on the back of my neck and insisted that I see my doctor immediately. So off I went to Dr. Charles Steinberg (for the first time in five years), carrying along my friend, the tick.

While I was about it, I had a full physical examination. My doctor was sure the tick had done me no harm, but that was the only good news.

The doctor's first grim pronouncement was that my diets were not working. That came as no surprise—at the time I wasn't even on a diet. I weighed three hundred pounds, far too much even for my height of five feet eleven inches. I had tried many diets in the past, but most of them had been notable only for their brevity.

His second point, delivered after the test results were in, was the real shocker. My cholesterol count was a dangerously high 324 and my blood sugar was soaring. If I didn't lower these levels, as well as my weight, he warned, *I wouldn't live to see my children grow up.*

I had been fighting my weight for years, and I knew that my health was not as good as it should have been, but until that moment I had no idea how serious my situation was. I was shaken.

I began immediately to change my eating habits and my lifestyle. I knew I couldn't wait for tomorrow. I might drop dead tomorrow.

VICTORY OVER ME

For most of my adult life I have been a compulsive eater. *I am still a compulsive eater, but I am now in remission and in one year I lost over one hundred pounds and have kept it off.* That remission has been more satisfying to me than all my years of out-of-control eating, all my obsessions with eating the best and the most, all the false victories won by controlling my food and your food and everybody's food. ("Controlling" food, as any compulsive eater knows, means eating it all.)

Compulsive eating is not a bad habit, it is a disease. But unlike some other diseases, compulsive eating doesn't go into remission by itself. I decided that I could take control of this disease, and in a split second I made the decision to conquer it. I did not decide that I would kick the compulsion "soon" or "tomorrow." I leapt into a new life-style immediately.

I can report that my new program worked. My wife, Susan, says, "I've got my old guy back." When we first met, she thought I was a hunk. In time I became a chunk, but now I'm a hunk once more. She tells me that I'm fun to live with again. My sense of humor had disappeared when my eating was out of control—I was angry at myself and it spilled over onto the people around me. I was sneaky, too, as all compulsive eaters are when they try to keep their binges a secret. Now I'm neither.

How This Program Can Help You

Being in the food business, I never found it easy to eat moderately. I was and am surrounded all day by enough temptation to defeat any mortal. But where once I tasted everything to test its quality, now I only sniff. I'm a genius at snorting cookies and cakes—a few good whiffs can tell me their ingredients, their sweetness, and their degree of doneness. What is more, I enjoy sniffing. It isn't the same as eating, but it will do. And when a particular product needs to be tasted, I call in my official tasters, my daughters Katherine and Elizabeth and my wife, Susan.

Sure, I would prefer the old way, but a compulsive person can't afford preferences. If you are a compulsive eater you are eating yourself to death—death by overweight or death by cholesterol or a combination of both.

A WAY OUT

Are you a compulsive eater, a CE?

Do you feel powerless because you realize that diets and willpower are not enough to make you lose weight? Do you see yourself over-eating not because you are over-hungry, but because you can't seem to help yourself?

Have you lost weight (again and again) and then watched with a feeling of helplessness as you gained it all back, and more besides? Do you eat more food than you need, more food than you really want? Do you eat because you are tense or angry or disappointed? Do you eat food just because it's there? Do you see yourself doing all these things, and yet do you deny to yourself and everyone else that eating is a problem for you?

If you answered yes to these questions, you have a lot of company.

"Compulsive eating" is a broad term. Your problem may be a lot less serious than mine, but it isn't likely to go away by itself. Maybe you are not in my league as a compulsive eater. Maybe you are fighting ten stubborn pounds instead of one hundred and you are out of control sometimes but not all the time. Thank your lucky stars, but don't put down this book! My experiences, my methods, and my delicious recipes will give you the help you need to lose weight.

I was chronically overweight, my blood sugar was elevated, my cholesterol level was life threatening, and I wasted my time and energy tracking down food and devouring it. But now my weight and blood sugar are normal, my cholesterol numbers are better than normal, and I enjoy my life. It is possible to change! I did it and I am still going strong. This book will tell you *how* I did it and how you can do it.

I know that most people suffering, as I was, from overweight and elevated cholesterol levels simply *have not found a successful method of controlling their compulsive eating*. I know this because until I worked out my own program, my compulsion had been stronger than every diet and behavior-modification program I had encountered.

If I could conquer my eating problems, living daily in the world of food, making my living from food, surrounded as I am by the world's finest chocolate, butter, pastries, ice cream, and cookies, then you can conquer yours, too.

These three elements make up my approach:
- cholesterol modification
- control of compulsive eating
- fine cooking

Together they add up to weight loss.

Cholesterol modification is the cornerstone of my program. I changed the foods I ate because I had to lower my cholesterol levels. I began to concentrate on foods that were medically approved for a cholesterol-free, low-fat diet and to eliminate those that were high in cholesterol and fat (see my food lists, chapter 6). It was as simple as that. What a delight to realize that relatively few foods were forbidden.

Control of compulsive eating is a very close second to cholestoral modification in importance (maybe they are tied for first). If you are a CE, this book will help you to understand your compulsion and will give you strategies for keeping it in check. Even if you are not a CE you will find the strategies tremendously useful.

Fine cooking is the natural center of my program. When I learned that I had to lower my cholesterol, one of the first new foods I tried was oat bran breakfast cereal. As I put some in a bowl and poured in the skim milk, I thought I saw the whole thing turn to cement before my eyes. I realized that I couldn't live out a life sentence of eating the usual "healthy," bland food prescribed for lowering cholesterol and losing weight. I knew I could do better. I have spent my adult life in the food business and superb food is my passion. I decided to devote my energy and my expertise to developing recipes that were based on the most healthful foods available while meeting my personal standards of excellence. The recipes that I produced and that I share with you in this book are delicious and I guarantee they work.

WHERE TO FIND IT ALL

In chapter 2, I talk about how I lived with an eating compulsion for many years. I share all my stories with you, even the embarrassing ones. Food addiction was the strongest force in my life, as it may be in yours. I had many experiences that only another compulsive eater could understand, but that anyone stuggling to lose weight can learn from.

Chapter 3 recounts my rides up and down on the diet seesaw. Before I worked out this program, I was "on a diet" more times than I care to count: so much for the usefulness of diets.

In chapter 4, I explain how you can begin to control your food addiction by avoiding certain foods that trigger your overeating and cause you to fail on any diet. Eliminating your triggers will give you extra strength in your battle against bingeing on and "abusing" food—your addictive substance.

Chapter 5 explains the importance of what you eat to cholesterol modification and shows how weight loss and lowered cholesterol are interdependent. In this chapter I tell you how I came to include oat bran in my new, healthier way of eating, with great success (although it wasn't love at first taste). I introduce a simple checklist of food variables so that you can evaluate any recipe in terms of its healthful—and harmful—ingredients.

Chapter 6 presents my delicious weight-loss program—let's not call it a diet! Based on the Yes list and No list of foods, you will tailor meals that meet your needs and suit your tastes. The principles work and *you will not feel deprived on this delicious program—you will feel satisfied and delighted.*

Chapter 7 explains a personal exercise agenda and how it has helped me to keep my compulsion in check. Some kind of regular exercise is an essential part of this program. *Exercise helps you burn up calories, alleviates stress, and helps lower harmful cholesterol levels.* And there is this extra benefit: when you make a commitment to keep yourself moving with some kind of exercise that fits your life-style, you strengthen your control over your own life. The more disciplined you become, the better you will feel about yourself.

In chapter 8, I tell you about the importance of keeping a food journal. When you record everything you eat, as well as every food temptation you resist, *you learn how to monitor your compulsion.* From there it is a short step to changing your patterns and moving away from compulsive eating. Chapter 8 is packed with strategies for you to use against your compulsion. It tells you how *food fallbacks* can keep you from high-cholesterol, high-calorie binges. It explains how you can eat comforting *bridge foods* to tide you over compulsive cravings. Here is a chapter to lean on when you accomplish your behavioral change from compulsive eater to healthy eater.

Chapter 9 will help you choose delicious and satisfying food to eat no matter where you are: in restaurants, at parties, and even at sports events and while traveling. It gives you tips for dealing with the outside world (waiters, chefs, hostesses, and guests) and with your own doubts.

Chapter 10 takes you into my kitchen. Using this chapter, you can prepare delicious, filling, satisfying dishes. I don't give you dull,

How This Program Can Help You

uninspired diet-book recipes guaranteed to turn you off the book and into the nearest pizzeria. The recipes I have created for this book involve the best ingredients prepared and served simply and imaginatively. I haven't lowered the standards I set for cuisine way back when I was a *cuisinier* in France's world-famous Restaurant Troisgros.

Following the guidelines in this book, you will take control of your life and you will live better and eat better! You will find that this is truly a life-changing, life-enhancing, pleasurable program.

Chapter Two

My Life as a Compulsive Eater

I really don't know what made me a compulsive eater, but I used to blame all my problems on my fat cells. If the medical research is correct, fat people have more and bigger fat cells than thin people have. Logically, this would make it impossible for me to lose weight and keep it off. I believed that I had lots of big, juicy fat cells, while skinny people had just a few little, skinny fat cells, and that my fat cells were screaming "feed us, feed us!" all the time. It was probably all genetic, and because I was born with those fat cells, I was stuck with them. In other words, my weight is not my fault, so please pass the ice cream.

For a long time I used the fat-cell theory as a crutch: I leaned on it and didn't bother to change my eating behavior. I don't do that anymore. I don't discount the theory, but I don't rely on it either, and fat cells or no fat cells, I have been able to lose weight.

My mother tells me that when I was a baby she tied a bagel to my crib because when I gnawed on it, I stopped crying. Other kids got a rattle but that didn't work for me, so I got a bagel. "Pacifiers weren't allowed in those days," my mother recalls. "There was no demand feeding. I didn't have a lot of leeway, but nobody said I couldn't give you a bagel." Very early on, I learned that eating calmed me down. (My Italian friends tell me they were given a type of pretzel called a *taralle* to keep them happy.)

I became a chubby toddler and then a husky boy. I remember always thinking of myself as heavier than the other kids. I never considered myself to be of normal weight.

The dissolution of my parents' marriage when I was three added stress to my early childhood, and food was always there to smooth things out. I wonder how many compulsive eaters are children of divorced or troubled families, how many are people who experienced emotional trauma. I think this kind of addiction has to be compensatory in a way, with food taking the place of some security that a child misses. Even in relatively happy families, food can become the symbol of comfort when a child experiences stress.

When my stepfather joined us (I was six at the time) he brought his own frenzied attitude toward meals. Eating was a major preoccupation in our new family—I remember great parties in our Princeton, New Jersey, home, with corned beef and rolled beef and pastrami. And I also remember a strong feeling of competition. I felt that I had to protect my own food or it wouldn't be there in the morning. When my mother served dinner, she never passed platters of food—she knew they wouldn't make it around the table. We all got individual dinner plates, filled in the kitchen.

Most mothers did their food shopping once a week. My mother went food shopping every day—she had to. She would fill the car and bring her bundles home, but half the time the food never made it into the refrigerator because my brother, Bill, and I got to it first and devoured it or buried it in our own secret hiding places.

No storage place was sacred in our kitchen, and the freezer was especially tempting. We debunked the commonly held belief that a freezer was used to store food for long periods of time, as we devoured frozen candy bars and cake. Sometimes we showed restraint when my mother wrote on the boxes: "Don't eat this! Dinner party!"

THE EATING SICKNESS

Our local supermarket sold its steaks and chops in packages of three, so my mother would buy three packages of pork chops for her family of four, serving each of us two chops at dinner. The ninth chop sat in the middle of the table, beckoning the fastest eater. Those dinners were Olympic sprints, and to the victor went the extra chop. Deep in the soul of every compulsive eater, there is a demon urging: "Eat faster! They're gaining on you!"

One evening, my brother and my stepfather finished dinner in a dead heat and went for the extra pork chop. Bill's fork wildly speared the chop, and at the same instant, my stepfather's fork wildly speared my brother's hand. I remember vividly my brother's howls and my stepfather's distress. Amid all this chaos, I reached over and snatched the chop.

We ate fast and we talked fast; at the dinner table we went for speed and volume. We were so eager to get to the next portion that we barely tasted what we were eating and whatever hit the table was devoured as if hit by a buzz saw. We didn't think of food as being good or bad—it was simply either enough or not enough.

We didn't restrict our hysteria to the family dining room or even to Princeton, New Jersey. One summer, the whole family traveled to Switzerland, and early in the trip we stopped at a lovely country inn and sat down to dinner. No sooner had the waiter put the food on our plates than it was gone—we inhaled it in the blink of an eye. Another waiter came by with the gravy and there was nothing to put it on. A very proper family at the next table stared at us in horror.

At home, between meals, we played games to hide our food consumption from each other. One of them was "Layering the Cookies": any one of us could eat most of a box of cookies and rearrange the layers as he proceeded, so that the box always appeared to be full.

Another routine was called "The Bottom, Side, Top Theory of Eating a Chocolate Cake." This was my specialty. If I opened the refrigerator and saw a big, fudgy, gooey chocolate cake, the game began. I would stare at the cake, filled with longing, and finally say to myself: "If I just take a little off the bottom, nobody will notice. Besides, how many calories can there be in the bottom?" So I would eat the bottom. Then I would say: "Maybe I should just eat the sides to even out the cake, now that I've eaten the bottom. How many calories can there be in the sides?" Of course I would move to the top of the cake, eat that, and then find there was nothing left but the middle. I would have no choice but to eat the middle, because I didn't want to leave any evidence. Besides, how many calories could there be in the middle? So there I was, fat and full of chocolate. I had finished the entire cake without eating any calories. For me, denial began at an early age.

One of our favorite family activities was "stopping," something you do only in the suburbs, where driving is a way of life. It goes like this: You are on your way from Nassau County to Suffolk County, but you pass a Dairy Queen stand and before you know it, the car has pulled in and stopped. You drive a few more miles and then, as if by magic, the car stops at a pizza place. Before your trip is over, you have stopped ten times, and every stop just seemed to happen automatically. A fifteen-minute trip, done this way, could take hours.

By the sixth grade I had become self-conscious about my weight, and my school's weighing policy didn't make me feel any better. Twice a year, the school nurse would go from room to room, rolling her portable scale along with her, and weigh each child. Then, in a thundering voice, she would call out his or her weight for an assistant to write down in the record book—and so that all the world could hear it. We never knew when the day of reckoning would come. Had I expected the nurse's visit, I definitely would have cut school.

But I did the next best thing. One day, soon after Christmas vacation ended, I heard the ominous sound of a heavy scale being rolled down the long hall. It had started far away, but it was coming closer and closer. I jumped up and sprinted out of my classroom, down the corridor away from the advancing scale, and out the door. "Where are you going?" my teacher yelled. "I'm sick," I called over my shoulder. If our classroom had been on the second floor, I think I would have jumped out of the window.

But I wasn't ready to cut down on my eating. My brother, Bill, remembers that I pioneered the concept of the pillowcase as Halloween bag. The other kids in the neighborhood went trick-or-treating carrying paper bags, which would break, spilling out their contents. I dressed up as a hobo, slung a pillowcase over my shoulder, and had no breakage problems. And more important, I quadrupled the capacity of the ordinary candy sack. Pretty soon everyone in the neighborhood was using pillowcases.

On Halloween I would eat all my candy (and the other kids' candy, too) before I got home, because I knew that once I walked through my front door, someone would pounce on it. In the best competitive spirit, I ate infinitely more than I wanted.

I always wolfed down lots of sweets, especially Twinkies, Hostess cupcakes, and frozen Snickers bars. Even before I knew how to drive, I ate in the car where no one could bother me, and I hid all the wrappers under the seat. Once I learned to drive, I began to haunt the local Dairy Queen stand. I would buy a pint of vanilla ice cream and some hot fudge sauce and make my own sundae, because their sundaes weren't big enough. This presented a problem of logistics: how do you fit the fudge sauce into a one-pint container that is already packed to the brim with vanilla ice cream? My solution was brilliant. I bought two one-pint containers of ice cream. I transferred a bit of ice cream from the first to the second carton, and poured some sauce into the space I had made. I ate a little ice cream and poured in a little more sauce. Before long, eating and pouring, I had everything in the right proportions.

I was on a constant lookout for new treats. Whenever I went to the local deli or grocery store, I headed straight for the candy rack and the ice-cream freezer to purchase the latest arrivals. I told myself that I would be in the food business when I grew up, and it wasn't too early to start tasting. I had a very good taste memory and I stored a lot in my memory bank. I always loved ice cream, and I

My Life as a Compulsive Eater

discovered Haagen Dazs long before most other people did. Getting there first is important to a compulsive eater.

Eating the most is important, too. Bill remembers one day at summer camp when he was searching for me. He asked everyone in my bunk where David was, but he got only blank looks in return. Finally one of my bunkmates said: "Oh, you must mean Meatball," and sent him off in the right direction. I had broken the camp record for eating meatballs (I forget how many) and no one called me by my given name after that triumph. I was the meatball champ.

One summer Bill went away to camp without me and he really missed the family. He decided to present me and our stepfather with a fabulous gift: every single day he bought one candy bar from the canteen and stashed it away in his duffle bag, saving the entire summer's collection for us. But at the end of the summer he sadly found that some mice had gotten to the candy first—he had nothing to bring home. If he had made a tray or a belt in the crafts shop, I guess he wouldn't have been so disappointed, but those would have been gifts for another family. For us, a gift of food was the best proof of love.

I was a good athlete, and was on the high school wrestling team when I was sixteen. I had to be weighed the day before every match, and if I exceeded the limit I couldn't wrestle. I always made the weight because I was careful not to overeat enough to ruin my chances to compete. But then I found myself with twenty-four hours before wrestling, when I could gain as much as I liked and no one would be the wiser. So after being weighed at school I would come home and gorge myself on six Twinkies and a six-pack of soda.

I loved dining with my family at Princeton's Nassau Inn when that restaurant offered its excellent roast beef buffets. Those buffets seemed especially wonderful to me because the food was unlimited and no one ever told me to stop eating.

I would walk up to the carver and ask for two or three ribs of beef, not the usual thin "English slice." Ecstatically, I would carry the huge hunk of meat back to my table and gnaw at it like a carnivorous animal. And when I finished the first portion, I would go back for more.

I only ate the "good stuff" on the buffet table—the roast beef, shrimp, lobster, and fried chicken. I didn't bother with the things I considered "filler," like the popovers, potatoes, bread, salad, or vegetables. My first rule of buffet management was: never worry about eating a balanced meal.

I soon came to feel that the restaurant staff knew me and that when I walked in the door there was a tense moment at the serving station. Nut cases like me, who didn't play by the rules and eat reasonable portions with popovers, threw the management's profit percentages out of whack.

My love of roast beef was nurtured both at the Nassau Inn and in my grandmother's kitchen. For years my gastronomic high point was coming into New York City to visit my grandmother, a great cook who served prime ribs of beef topped with a crusty layer of fat. I loved to open the oven and cut off a piece of the crispy, crunchy crust, oozing melted fat, and eat that. I'm amazed when I hear thin people talk fondly about their mothers' or grandmothers' salads or Brussels sprouts. For me, it is the crisp fat enrobing a prime rib roast that memories are made of.

These visits to Grandma's house had another benefit. I usually excused myself from the family early in the afternoon and walked over to Greenberg's, the famous New York bakery, where the aroma of butter and warm caramel put me into a semi-trance. My mother liked to shop there too. She would buy pounds of the yeasty, sugary pastries called *schnecken*, transport them home, and freeze them (that is, freeze what had survived the journey). Most families would have defrosted them over time in small amounts—maybe warming them in the oven to release their cinnamon fragrance—and then would have gathered at the kitchen table to enjoy them as a leisurely treat. Not us! We didn't bother to defrost the pastries or even to sit down. My favorite pastry always has been frozen Greenberg's schnecken, eaten standing up, in front of an open freezer door.

My Life as a Compulsive Eater

I returned to Greenberg's when I was a sophomore at New York University, older but not much wiser. I had an apartment on East Twelfth Street and Greenberg's had a shop on East Eighth Street. This was in 1968, at the height of student unrest, but my energy went into overeating, not revolution. Every day I passed the shop on my way to class—or rather, I never passed the shop by. I always stopped in and bought a few schnecken, as well as other treats.

I spent enough time in Greenberg's to become friendly with the saleswomen. Every morning I breakfasted there and every evening, after school, I bought a snack for immediate consumption (to "take the edge off" my appetite), plus a little something to keep for after dinner.

I soon went from being in good shape (having been on Denison University's lacrosse team the year before) to being overweight. Actually, I gained about thirty pounds during the fall semester at NYU-Greenberg's.

I knew where the trouble lay. So I walked into the bakery and told my friends, the saleswomen, that I was beginning a diet. "If I come in here and ask for something," I said firmly, "don't give it to me! Just say, 'No, David, go away,' and I will go away."

It became a game. I would drop by every morning and say: "I'll take a dozen schnecken and a half-pound of cookies and a babka," and they would say, "No, David, go away."

I lost thirty pounds. In addition to foregoing pastries, I changed my dinner habits. I stopped dining on thick steaks and ate roast chicken instead, and I tried to avoid other fattening foods. I was fine until one frosty February night, when, exhausted from studying, I fell victim to a Greenberg's attack.

Fortunately it was very late and I knew the shop had closed hours before. I told myself the craving would pass and I fell into a restless sleep. But when I awoke in the morning I felt even worse.

I got dressed and raced to Greenberg's.

"Hi," I said. "I'll take a dozen schnecken and a half-pound of cookies and a babka."

"No, David," said the women. "Go away."

Through clenched teeth I said, "Give me the schnecken."

"Go away," they answered.

I hissed: "Give me the schnecken or I'll steal them." I was like a drug addict robbing a store. The saleswomen realized that I was deadly serious and they sold me the pastries. I ran back to my apartment and ate myself sick. And it wouldn't be the last time.

I left NYU and temptation, and graduated from SUNY-Old Westbury (a place where, at that time, I couldn't seem to find anything very interesting to eat). After a year spent remodeling brownstones and working as a short-order cook in a New York coffee shop, I entered Brooklyn Law School.

By day, I was a dutiful son, studying law to please my parents. By night, I was a budding chef, studying at the Statler Restaurant School at New York City Community College. (This pleased my parents too. They knew that the food business had intrigued me all my life.)

Every summer vacation for five years I had visited France, making myself known and, I hoped, indispensable to the Restaurant Troisgros in Roanne. Sure enough, after my law school graduation in 1975, the Troisgros brothers hired me as *commis* and soon promoted me to *cuisinier*, an unheard-of position for an American. I spent six months at Troisgros, working fourteen to eighteen hours a day, usually seven days a week.

I had discovered Troisgros by chance one summer when I was in Marseille, choosing whether I wanted to see Snowflake, the white gorilla at the Barcelona zoo, or whether I wanted to have a three-star meal. I decided on the meal, and to this day I have yet to see Snowflake. My budget was tight and it was more economical for me to drive five hours to Troisgros than to eat at a closer, more expensive restaurant, so that is what I did. I fell in love with the restaurant when I ate that first meal.

When I came back home I worked briefly for a New York law firm but I soon realized that my heart was in the food business. I set up a company called Saucier that produced and marketed frozen sauce concentrates. The company didn't really take off, which is a shame because the product was excellent. So I moved from sauces to cookies, with enormous success, and I opened first one, then another New York restaurant. Along the way I wrote *Cooking the Nouvelle Cuisine in America* with Michèle Urvater.

I had worked for Restaurant Troisgros and I had discovered the joys of the *Guide Michelin* and its star system. This led me to another kind of compulsive eating, even more intense than the one I had grown up with at Dairy Queen and Greenberg's.

THE STAR SYSTEM

People have goals. Some people want to climb Mount Everest and some people want to run the New York City Marathon. My goal was considerably more compulsive: to eat the best food this world had to offer. I believed that kind of food was to be had in France's three-star restaurants. Restaurant Troisgros, where I was lucky enough to work, is one of the few restaurants that the *Guide Michelin* honors with a three-star rating.

This guide to fine hotels and restaurants was created in 1900 by the Michelin tire company as a way to encourage motorists to drive more (and buy more tires). Over the years it has become a bible to gastronomes the world over. Any establishment listed in the guide must meet certain standards determined by the Michelin board of review. The book lists hotels and restaurants that are good bargains, and it also has the star system.

Michelin lists about 550 one-star restaurants and about seventy two-star restaurants, as well as those few three-star establishments it considers to be the epitome of fine food preparation and service. French chefs will dedicate their lives to attaining a three-star rating and will go to extremes to keep it.

Whenever I took a vacation, I didn't consider where in the world I might go or what new experience I might seek. I didn't go to Outward Bound, or climb a mountain, or shoot the rapids. My only plans dealt with when I could leave for France and how I could make the connections to eat at the most three-star restaurants in the shortest possible time.

THE EATING SICKNESS

I did it for years, starting in the late 1960s and going on through the early 1980s. I would travel to France and make the circuit, racing from restaurant to restaurant, sometimes eating at two places in one day. I can tell you the distances between three-star restaurants more easily than I can clock a trip from Manhattan to New Jersey or Long Island.

I set out to eat at every three-star restaurant, and by 1981 I had accomplished this goal. Then Michelin added some new ones and took off a few, which threw me a little out of sync.

What made three-star restaurants so important to me as a compulsive eater? These places played directly into my obsession with food and overeating. They gave legitimacy to my excess and total lack of control.

The name of the game was overkill. I would start lunch at 12:00 and finish somewhere between 4:00 and 5:00 P.M., having polished off seven courses of food, two bottles of wine, ten desserts, and Cognac or Armagnac. A half hour later, the phenomenon I knew as the "three-star high" would descend on me. This was the most incredible feeling I had ever experienced. I knew I had eaten as well as anybody had ever eaten, and all was right with the world. But my high never lasted long enough. The food and drink would catch up with me in a battering wave of nausea and exhaustion.

The famous Restaurant Pyramide was one of my favorite spots for overindulging because of its unique location: after my meal, I could stumble to the riverbank and collapse surrounded by beautiful scenery.

Just to put this in perspective, in 1973, about the time I was stalking restaurants like a big-game hunter, you could do yourself in at Troisgros for 98 francs, or $18.00, plus 20 francs, or $3.50, for each bottle of wine. For this reasonable sum you were served a seemingly endless progression of courses, culminating in the grand dessert.

In the 1970s, dessert was carried to ridiculous extremes, even in my terms. One day I was dining at Restaurant Chapel and two waiters brought over a huge platter that had fifteen different pies and fruit pastries, and that was just the start. After that they came over with a tray of thirty chocolate desserts—cakes and logs and mousses and truffles. Then came twelve different ice creams, and finally, candies. I didn't eat it all, but it defined my craziness. It offered total gluttony.

The chefs were all too eager to bury a willing tourist under mountains of food. If an American had traveled thousands of miles for lunch or dinner, these chefs were delighted to feed that person's fantasy. Besides, it was excellent promotion. The tourist would return home and tell his friends: "You won't believe that I had twenty-seven desserts at Troisgros!"

A few people go to these restaurants to eat sparingly. The question is, why don't they go someplace where they can eat for less money? Most people go to three-star restaurants to *eat*. They don't go to be seen or to sit in the status banquette. And compulsive people go for the experience of eating it all. They need to feel: "I conquered it."

In terms of my weight, each trip to France meant a gain of two pounds a day. If I stayed seven days, I gained fourteen pounds. But I was counting stars, not pounds. When I planned a seven-day trip, I counted the number of stars "consumed" per meal. Technically, the maximum that can be done is six per day, or forty-two stars in a week, but I don't think anyone on earth is capable of that. However, I could eat meals totaling thirty stars in a seven-day trip if I occasionally ate two three-star meals in a single day.

Early in my quest, I was driving with my then-current girlfriend from lunch at Troisgros to dinner at Bocuse. We had left our first meal about 4:30 and were driving insanely to reach the second restaurant, even though I was ill and nauseous from overindulging at lunch. I pulled the car over to the side of the road and began laughing hysterically. We had eaten enough to keep us alive for two weeks, and here we were, racing to the next meal, which we couldn't possibly finish.

We canceled the dinner and rescheduled it for the next day, but all night long I suffered pangs of anxiety because I had missed a three-star meal. Maybe they had served something that they would never serve again! I couldn't have eaten it anyway—or could I? Many times before I had "worked through" the nausea and had just kept on chewing. I have some fond memories of "eating myself to death" almost the way it was done in the classic French film, *Le Grande Bouffe*.

And the scary part, the part that reminds me of my mortality, is that if I am not careful, I think I have it in me to do it all over again.

THE ENEMY WITHIN

Like all compulsive people, I fought a constant battle against my addiction. Sometimes I won, but I was never able to stay victorious for very long. I remember that my wife, Susan, and I traveled from Italy to France when we were engaged. I was a perfectly reasonable eater in Italy—the Italians are wonderful cooks and are sensible about what they serve you. But as soon as I got to France I began to lose control.

On this particular day, we had a two-star lunch, and Susan didn't want any dinner. Nevertheless we continued on to Restaurant Pic in Valence, where I expressed interest in the Menu Rabelais, a ten-course tasting menu. The captain told me it could only be prepared for two people, and, unfortunately, Susan wasn't having any. Undaunted, I announced: "I will take it for two."

I was now looking at Susan's dinner plus mine: twenty courses and dessert. I was ecstatic because I was in a three-star restaurant *eating double* and doing it without being a pig—I was just eating my fiancée's food.

I merrily devoured the first two courses as they arrived, with Susan keeping me company but not eating a bite. Then the third course was served. It was a whole fresh truffle wrapped in fois gras, then wrapped in pastry, and then baked over a wood fire. I bit into my truffle and it was magnificent. I said to Susan: "I'm going to enjoy your truffle enormously." That tempted her, and she decided to taste it. It was so delicious that she ate the whole thing.

I was deeply in love with Susan, but at that moment I was filled with disbelief, disappointment, and rage. That was *my* truffle she was eating! I wanted to divorce her right there, and we weren't even married yet!

THE LOCAL STAR SYSTEM

While France remains a shrine to overeating, the United States also has a lot to offer. The major compulsive eaters of the world zero in on Kansas City, Missouri, because it has an inordinate amount of delicious junk food.

I liked the Kansas City barbecue restaurants because even at my heaviest, I was one of their thinnest patrons. These places are furnished very simply with counters and high round stools. Many a customer's rear end takes up two stools. When I was starting David's Cookies I went to St. Louis to look at an oven I was interested in buying. My business concluded, I had a choice: Did I go home to New York City or go the other way, to Kansas City to have dinner at the famous Arthur Bryant's? Calvin Trillin, one of my favorite food writers, had called Arthur Bryant's the greatest restaurant in the world. I immediately hopped a plane for Kansas City. I arrived at about six in the evening and called the restaurant.

"How late are you open?" I asked.

"Open? We close at six," was the reply.

To me, this was the ultimate definition of chutzpah: a restaurant that closed for dinner!

I was told that Bryant's would open at nine in the morning, and the next morning I was there. You would think it was a little early for barbecued ribs, but I nevertheless had to get in line behind twenty other early birds. As I waited I got hungrier and more frantic, so that when my turn came I ordered and ate thirty dollars' worth of barbecue for breakfast.

THE EATING SICKNESS

The next time I visited Kansas City, Larry "Fats" Goldberg, a friend of Trillin's, took me around the circuit. This meant going to seven places for dinner in one night: Bryant's, Gates's, Chicken Betty's, Chicken Sally's, Grandma's, and Stroud's. Best of all, there was Slow Richard's.

Slow Richard started as a slicer at Bryant's (a very slow slicer) and then opened his own place. He used to pick up the meat with one hand, put in on a slice of white bread, paint it with sauce using a paintbrush, take a pile of greasy French fries with his hand, put them on top of the sauce, and cover them with another slice of bread. It was out of this world. Calvin Trillin believed that the reason the meat tasted so good was that Slow Richard had a particular enzyme in his hands that flavored it.

There was always a long line of people waiting for Richard's spectacular barbecue. When Fats and I walked into his restaurant, he would give us portions of the burnt ends—the crusty part that falls off when you slice the meat—which to me are heaven. We would also have a couple of sandwiches and several pounds of ribs, and this was only one of our seven meals. Stroud's was the last of the seven restaurants, where we went for fried chicken and biscuits. It is a measure of our obsession that their slogan, "We choke our own chickens," didn't diminish our appetites.

New Haven, Connecticut, is another mecca for compulsive eaters, who consider it the pizza capital of the United States. I used to drive up from New York for a snack, doing the ninety miles very quickly to get to a place called Sally's on South Wooster Street. Sally was an old, anorexic-looking man who made fantastic thin-crust pizzas. Unfortunately, he smoked over the pizzas, so I took my business elsewhere.

I walked down the street to a place called Pepe's, where they made an incredibly delicious white-clam pizza. After discovering Pepe's, I went through a phase of traveling to New Haven just to eat the white-clam pizza. Then, for about a year, I paid a conductor on the New Haven Line to pick up pizzas at Pepe's and bring them to New York, where I would meet the train. Everybody who goes to

Yale knows about the pizza places, and if they don't, maybe they shouldn't have gotten into Yale in the first place.

There are small restaurants like this all over the country, and they offer two challenges to the compulsive eater. One, he has to discover them, and two, he has to conquer them by eating himself into the ground.

THE COMPULSIVE EATER'S WORLD

There are degrees of compulsive eating. Some people never reach a weight of 313 pounds, as I briefly did. They let themselves go to a certain point and then they crash diet back down again. Yet they are compulsive: when they binge, they are totally out of control. Some eaters are compulsive only once in a while, perhaps with certain foods that have proven to be poison to them in terms of self-control. They keep their compulsion in the closet most of the time.

My definition of compulsive eating is a wide one, encompassing a broad spectrum of people. For instance, a good friend of mine, an attractive young mother of two, lives in daily fear of her compulsion, even though her weight has not fluctuated by more than three pounds in the past ten years! When she does gain those three pounds now and again, she is frightened that she will lose all control and balloon up to two hundred pounds—a weight she has never come close to.

But in contrast to my friend is the woman who owns clothing in several sizes: thin, medium, and fat. She has gained and lost weight countless times and the only solution she knows to this problem is to be prepared in terms of wardrobe. When it comes to controlling her weight and her eating, she feels totally hopeless. Like most compulsive eaters, this woman cannot leave food alone—if it is there, she feels she must eat it. She remembers completing a six-week diet and immediately sitting in a corner with a large bag of potato chips and finishing it down to the last crumb.

Contrary to myth, most compulsive eaters are not hungry for breakfast. Food addicts generally do their major eating between five and ten at night. Then they go to bed for a while, before they get up and raid the refrigerator. Very few of them wake up each morning and eat a loaf of white bread, a pound of bacon, and a dozen eggs.

There are many compulsive eaters whom you never see eating, although sometimes these people are caught in the act. A friend told me of the time she baked a luscious lemon meringue pie to serve at a dinner party. She was shocked when she walked into her kitchen between courses and found one of her guests devouring the dessert!

When I decided to do myself in, I usually didn't try to hide it. However, most people don't overeat in front of a spouse, and I was no exception. Susan could not figure out when or where I binged. What she didn't see was me out on the streets of New York, a walking delicatessen, with candy bars in my pocket and a hot dog in each hand.

You won't see many compulsive eaters gorging themselves at restaurants or parties. They don't order two steaks and three lobsters—in fact, they don't order any more food than the average person does. All around the compulsive eater are people who wonder how someone who eats so little has gotten so fat. But a compulsive eater is like someone on an intravenous feeding tube—there is a continuous supply of food. The feeding never stops.

Sometimes food addicts try to outsmart their compulsion, only to find the compulsion is smarter than they are. One woman totally emptied her apartment of food when she began a crash diet, but she kept the keys to a neighbor's apartment. One day, in desperation, she emptied his refrigerator while he was at work.

CEs can overeat unobtrusively at a restaurant or family dinner because they eat faster than normal eaters. They quietly move into seconds, or extra bites from their spouse's plate. I always ate much faster than Susan, anticipating that wonderful moment when she would ask: "Are you still hungry? Do you want some of mine?" I felt it was my right to take food from her plate. Of course I had my own food; that was a given. Susan's was a bonus. I knew I was getting desperate when I started working on my children's plates.

Eating fast becomes an ingrained habit for CEs and it is very difficult to break. People try all sorts of gimmicks to slow down: counting to fifty between bites, chewing each mouthful one hundred times, sipping water between mouthfuls of food, even eating with a programmed fork that flashes a green light for go and a red light for stop. None of these seems to work.

A compulsive eater doesn't eat fast and overeat because he or she enjoys food. *The idea is to control the food,* to make it all belong to him or her. A compulsive eater can't eat dinners family style: when a serving platter is passed around the table, a compulsive fights the urge to take every last morsel. Unable to grab it all, he or she will take a normal portion and eat it fast enough to go back for more immediately.

A compulsive person can't share food—I know families who buy separate pint, quart, or even half-gallon containers of ice cream for each family member, and label them with the individual's names. When my eating was out of control, if anyone asked me to share my ice-cream cone I would sooner kill him than say yes.

I put a lot of energy into compulsive eating, and let me assure you, I was not alone. Each year, as I frantically toured France's three-star restaurants, I met the same people again and again. Later I met many of them at spas. For them, the spa circuit was the flip side of the restaurant circuit.

Many people who work in the food business are obsessed with food. The legendary Fernand Point, owner of La Pyramide, said that when he went to other restaurants, his first stop would be the kitchen. If he saw a skinny chef he woud leave, because he believed that a thin cook was incapable of preparing excellent food. However, if the restaurant had a good reputation, he would inquire if the chef had been fat in the past and had lost a great deal of weight.

But food obsession is not the same as love of fine food. I find that many food addicts eat not because they appreciate food, but because they feel unable to control the world around them. The only thing they can control is what they do or do not put into their mouths.

SHOPPING FOR CLOTHES

Buying clothes is a fairly normal part of life, but it can be agony for someone who is heavy.

Speaking for men, I know that the process involves going to a specialty store and pretty much taking what we can get. An obese man doesn't want to admit his size to anyone, so he asks the salesman for a size that won't humiliate him. Then the clothes come into the dressing room and go flying back out because they are too tight. The usual definition of salesperson—someone who asks you what you would like to see and then points you in the right direction—doesn't apply when a CE shops. A salesperson is someone who keeps throwing larger sizes at you.

When women are overweight they often try to skip shopping altogether. Pat, a clothing designer who owns several stores in the New York and Connecticut area, told me: "I sometimes don't see certain customers for months. That's when I know they have gained a lot of weight fast and are in hiding."

And her sales assistant added: "If a customer is overweight we both know that she is limited to bulky, oversize styles. Even if I find something that fits and flatters, it's hard to please someone who is unhappy about her figure before she even starts to try things on!"

ADJUSTING TO CHANGE

I've been at a fairly normal weight for some time now, but I have only just started to give or throw away my "fat clothes." I can't bear to part with them and I tell myself that I had better keep them a little while longer. Suppose I need something to polish the car?

Recently, when I needed a new pair of pants, I ventured into the strange territory of Bloomingdale's. I'm not heavy anymore, so I was able to choose clothes like a normal person, but I was still anxious. Thinking like the fat person I once was, I asked the salesman: "Do you have anything to fit me?" Did he? Everything in the store fit me! I walked into this football field of clothes with probably ten thousand pairs of pants that I could buy, and I didn't know what to do next. I used to buy any pair of pants that fit me in whatever lousy color there was. Now this guy told me that I could pick any pair of pants I wanted. I was in that store, suffering, *trying to deal with choices, for over three hours—something new to me*.

THE REAL WORLD

One thing that compulsive eaters don't let themselves experience is the feeling of hunger. I was never hungry—I was always eating something. I didn't differentiate between eating a meal and eating between meals, I just ate.

Hunger is a bewildering sensation and I can't say at this point that I enjoy it. Occasionally I will have a really busy day and not have time for lunch. Then I try to deal with this fascinating thing called hunger. I may be hungry for an hour, God forbid, before I get to have my dinner.

With different people, between-meal hunger has different effects. When Susan gets hungry, she gets edgy, and she says her blood sugar is down to her ankles. I tell her, "Go and get something to eat. I'm not talking to you until you get your blood sugar up."

Hunger makes me depressed. I feel sorry for myself because I have nothing to eat and who knows—I could starve to death. What if the bomb is dropped and I haven't eaten? Even today, if I saw a white flash in the sky and I knew we would all turn to sawdust in ten seconds, I'm afraid that my last thought probably would be: "Idiot, you didn't eat that pint of ice cream!" That's what I would go out with.

BREAKING THE COMPULSION

Perhaps I have made some of this obsessive behavior sound like fun—let me assure you, it was not. As a compulsive I was miserably unhappy with my weight, my appearance, and finally, my health. I felt guilty because I could not stick to diets, and I felt weak because my eating was irrational. But I was finally able to move from hating myself to hating the compulsion, and from there, to achieving self-control.

I have described my life of eating out of control, with all its attendant madness. If you recognize yourself in any of these stories, let me tell you how you, too, can change your behavior and your life.

I believe that if you are a compulsive eater, you will always be a compulsive eater. What is true for an alcoholic is true for you: although you can force your illness into remission, you cannot cure yourself totally. You will have to use a lot of your waking energy to control your food compulsion. If you truly want to exercise this control, you must do the following things:

1. Face the fact that for the foreseeable future you will avoid certain foods that you have depended. These foods act as triggers to your binges of overeating, and even one bite can lead to disaster (see chapter 4). Some of these foods might not be harmful to you if you could only eat them in moderation. But being a compulsive eater, you don't know what moderation is.
2. Follow a nutritionally sound food program like the one I give you in chapter 6. Using the recipes I have developed (and list in chapter 10), you will enjoy delicious, satisfying meals while you bring down your weight and your cholesterol count.
3. Keep a food journal (see chapter 8). The journal helps you monitor your eating compulsion and control it.
4. Exercise regularly (see chapter 7). If you do not exercise, my method will not work fully. And the benefits of exercise go beyond weight loss. Exercise improves your cholesterol levels, increases your fitness and strength, and alleviates stress.

This book will help you. It will give you a good idea how the mind of a compulsive person works and how to deal with your obsession on a daily basis. Every compulsive eater spends a lot of time and energy on the pursuit of food. You can channel that time and energy so that they will work for you, not against you.

Bear in mind that a compulsion is not logical. So if you want to cure your addiction, you can't just sit down and logically talk yourself out of it. Your compulsion is very, very difficult to reach. But if you follow my program, you can monitor it, outsmart it, and control it.

Chapter Three

Up and Down on the Diet Seesaw

Let me tell you why you have to *change your life* and not just go on a diet.

A diet is a quick fix—temporary by definition. A diet must end, and when it ends, you go back to eating the old way.

A diet doesn't teach you to change your behavior. When you accept what it tells you and follow its rules, you go from overeating to suffering. If you want to stay on your diet, you have to weigh and measure ounces, milligrams, and portion sizes. When you finish the diet, you haven't learned anything about normal eating. Then you are told to go on maintenance. What do you know about maintaining anything? You only know about overeating and suffering.

Many diets are simply gimmicks that prove, in the end, to be harmful. The ones that aren't harmful are often just plain silly. And even if you find a diet that makes some sense, you, the compulsive eater, will twist it to fit your needs. I know, because I went from one diet to another for many years and my compulsiveness wrecked them all.

The problem is not entirely in the diets themselves, although some of them are pretty ridiculous. Compulsive eating is an internal disease and diets are an attempt at an external cure. As long as somebody else is telling you to lose weight, you won't lose. *You have to take responsibility for your own eating habits and change your own behavior.*

If you eat compulsively, you eat when you don't need food and even when you don't enjoy food. Food is an addiction for a compulsive eater, a CE, the way alcohol is an addiction for an alcoholic. Most diets do not work because they ignore your addiction. But once you accept that fact, you will be able to attack your compulsion and conquer it. You need a program that makes sense for you as an *addictive personality*.

None of the diets I tried worked for me as a CE, yet I kept coming back for more. In my old, compulsive life, Monday often meant the start of a new diet. Many of these diets never made it to Tuesday. Here is the way I spent too many Mondays of my life. Maybe you'll recognize yourself in my story.

MONDAY—A NEW DIET BEGINS

I wake up in the morning feeling virtuous and have a cup of black coffee. I don't exercise and I don't eat breakfast. I had started my diet at 12:01 A.M. (probably after polishing off some ice cream one minute before midnight) and my resolve is strong.

By eleven in the morning I feel really good about myself because I haven't eaten anything for eleven hours. About noon, the thought of lunch crosses my mind, and I start fantasizing about fried chicken. Then I remind myself that I am on a diet and I have a meager lunch. I have been denying myself for twelve hours—so far, so good.

When 2:00 P.M. rolls around I start to feel sorry for myself; it has been a long time since I tasted anything good. I trudge along stoically for another two hours or so, but then, about 4:30, I start to weaken. As hunger overwhelms me, I put my powers of reason on hold and I tell myself that I simply must have something to "take the edge off." So I have something: a couple of candy bars and a few hot dogs.

Meanwhile, my wife is at home preparing a sensible meal for me, not knowing that somewhere between lunch and dinner, once again I have fallen into the abyss.

I come home to my supportive wife and I tell her what I think she should hear: I have been very good. I skipped breakfast and I ate hardly anything for lunch, and here I was eating her delicious diet dinner. (I don't mention the hot dogs and candy.)

After dinner, I go upstairs to read a book or watch television and I sink into depression. I think about starving myself all day and then bingeing at 4:30. Another diet shot! I feel that I am totally out of control. Almost in a trance, I shuffle down to the kitchen and eat everything I can lay my hands on. By 11:30 the feeding frenzy is over and I roll into bed. "Well, maybe next Monday," I tell myself and fall asleep.

DIETS I HAVE KNOWN

I must have started hundreds of diets. I had very little trouble starting them and I had less trouble ending them. Of course, they didn't all collapse on the first day. Some lasted weeks and one or two lasted months. I even lost weight on some of these diets. However, when the diet ended, I always regained every pound I lost, plus a few more.

I had a major problem with dieting because I wanted immediate results and if I didn't get them, my motivation dissolved. But I was accustomed to eating large quantities of food daily. When I began a diet, my body would have to work its way through days of the accumulated food I had eaten and was in the process of sluggishly digesting, before the diet took hold. All the food I had stuffed myself with wasn't going away overnight, so I often lost heart and many diets went away overnight.

Up and Down on the Diet Seesaw

The diet I relied on more than any other was the Drinking Man's Diet, or some variation of it. I think I was on and off this one thirty times in my life. It limited my intake of carbohydrates, but I could eat unlimited fat. If I ate three baked potatoes and some vegetables I would go over my carbohydrate limit, but I could stuff myself with pork chops, bacon, and foie gras to my heart's content. At least that was my interpretation of the rules. I often cut the carbohydrate allowance in half (a compulsive person has to do things better) while feasting on fifteen pork chops fried in butter for dinner. I was probably consuming seven thousand to ten thousand calories daily and hardly any of those came from carbohydrates.

It amazed me that I could eat the kind of food I ate on binges and still be on a diet. I would wake up and, despite my natural aversion to breakfast, eat four eggs and a half-pound of bacon. (I avoided orange juice and toast because of their carbohydrate content.) For lunch I had fried chicken—cutting into my carbohydrate allowance just a bit. Dinner would be a big steak or those pork chops, hold the potatoes and salad. I could drink all the wine I wanted to.

I remember two things about this diet: I found the food delicious, because I loved rich, highly marbled meat and fried chicken; and it helped me get crazier than I already was. Somehow the Drinking Man's Diet legitimized my ridiculous eating habits.

I managed to lose weight each time I went on this diet. Week one meant a weight loss of about ten pounds; after that it was two to four pounds a week. But this diet, like all diets, was self-limiting. For weeks I consumed my trigger foods in huge quantities every day—I was free to eat as much of them as I desired. But triggers have a dual effect: not only do you overeat the trigger foods, you also want to overeat lots of other things. For me, the point always came when the fifteen pork chops had to lead to the three pints of ice cream. That was the explosive moment the diet ended and I went back to binges that included carbohydrates. Of course I gained back every pound I had lost.

A lot of people thought such a high-protein, high-fat diet was fine, but in the midst of dieting I had my doubts. I would go to the supermarket and get a four-pound steak, and as I was putting it into my basket I would think, "Does it really make sense to eat this? Wouldn't I do better with a potato and some vegetables?" But the Drinking Man's Diet was similar to the Air Force Diet, which had the sanction of the U.S. government. Later, Dr. Robert C. Atkins offered another variation of it with his "Diet Revolution." Who could quarrel with those credentials?

I never stayed on this diet for more than two months at a time, but I often came back to it after I broke up with another diet. It helped tide me over.

A compulsive eater tries to do everything better than the next guy, and in this spirit I reduced the Drinking Man's Diet down to its essence. For a while I decided to live only on wine for lunch and dinner. As it happens, I lost a lot of weight on that variation of my old standby. Obviously, I wasn't too lucid while I was losing it. I gave up this program pretty quickly.

I also got around to the Grapefruit Diet, which was very popular for a while. It involved eating half a grapefruit before every meal—grapefruit before breakfast, grapefruit before lunch, grapefruit before dinner, and then starting all over again with grapefruit the next day. I'm afraid I just don't like grapefruit that much. The diet was a flop for me.

The Hot Fudge Sundae Diet promised to be one of my favorites, and I started it with lots of enthusiasm. I ate hot fudge sundaes for breakfast, lunch, dinner, and snacks. I wasn't allowed to eat anything else. I was in college when I was following this plan, and I didn't have much money, so I bought the cheapest ice cream I could find. Every other day I went to the supermarket and bought four half-gallons of vanilla, chocolate, and strawberry (I'm a purist when it comes to ice cream), along with some fudge sauce and whipped cream in a pressurized can. I decided to forego the cherries.

Up and Down on the Diet Seesaw

I had a bit of a problem with the breakfasts. I didn't care for breakfast in general, and somehow a small hot fudge sundae to start the day made me a little queasy. But I was a good sport.

For lunch I had a medium-sized hot fudge sundae, and for a snack I had a small one, like the one I had eaten for breakfast. Dinnertime came and I abandoned all pretense of civility. I simply flipped back the top of the ice cream carton and gazed into the crater left by breakfast, lunch, and snack. Then I filled it with a pool of fudge sauce and dove in.

I lived this way for just under one week and I gained ten pounds. I was on a massive sugar high all week.

I got off it the only way I knew how. I swung back to the Drinking Man's Diet and had fifteen pork chops for dinner Sunday night, but no dessert.

Another diet that appealed to me was the Popcorn Diet. This was one of several filler diets I encountered. It kept my stomach filled with something relatively harmless—popcorn. Satiation is a good way of handling compulsive eating: just fill yourself up with popcorn, or beans, or potatoes, or seltzer, and you won't want to eat anything more.

The trick here was to eat popcorn before every meal. I was on this diet for a full week before I reverted to the Drinking Man's Diet. Unfortunately, after the popcorn I was expected to count calories for the rest of my meals. As an active CE, I couldn't accept that rule.

I went on the Weight Watchers' Diet for three days and gave up because, again, I had to measure portions. Another problem was that I hated listening endlessly to other people's dietary problems at Weight Watchers' meetings. I couldn't stand the breast-beating. I guess I'm just not a group person.

Clearly, I am not a calorie counter, either. Calorie counting may work for some people, but I find that it tends to make CEs fixate on food even more than usual (if that is possible). I learned this on one of my spa vacations, where calories were listed for every item on the menu. If someone were restricted to, say, a thousand calories a day, he or she had to mix and match foods to arrive at that total. The good news was that everyone at the table got into the spirit of counting calories; the bad news was that they talked about food every waking moment. That week I could have sold David's Cookies for a thousand dollars a pound, if I only had the foresight to bring some along.

On one of my diets I tried the ultimate gimmick in calorie counting. I walked around carrying a little hand-held calculator programmed to add up the calories I consumed. I punched in everything I ate for breakfast, lunch, dinner, and snacks. One day, out of scientific curiosity, I decided not to record my meals and just to record the snacks. My nibbles added up to well over three thousand calories.

For a while I put myself on what I called the Bulk Diet. I decided to weigh everything I ate: an apple, a pint of ice cream, a steak. Liquids were the only exception. I counted the total number of pounds I put into my body every day to see if that number affected the total number of pounds I gained. I figured out that if I ate three pounds and metabolized two and a half pounds, then I shouldn't gain more than half a pound. It didn't work.

Some diets I encountered allow the dieter "on" days and "off" days. When you follow one of these on-again-off-again diets, your food intake will be controlled on certain days of the week and totally up to you on the other days. If you restrict yourself part of the time, you are allowed to binge the rest of the time. This concept goes against everything I understand about trigger foods. For me and for many other compulsive eaters, only one bite of a trigger food can cause out-of-control eating. It is very difficult to climb back up once you have fallen over the cliff, and I know I couldn't do it every few days.

Such diets remind me of a friend who has a cholesterol problem, but not a weight problem. Once a year he allows himself a big, juicy steak. He makes this steak dinner into a festive occasion, celebrating and having a wonderful time. I simply couldn't stop at one steak.

I never tried any of the "modified fasting" diets that allow you to drink one or all of your meals in the form of a high-protein mixture. A friend of mine who was on a modified fast described his day for me. He said: "For breakfast I drink a glass of the diet mix. Then I eat nothing until lunchtime, when I have one more glass. I eat nothing all afternoon, and then I come home from work. At dinnertime I sit down at the table, and for dinner *I eat three meals—breakfast, lunch, and dinner!*" My friend has gained weight on this diet.

The only diet that ever worked for me is one I call the Exhaustion Diet. This came about by chance when I was toiling sixteen to eighteen hours a day at Restaurant Troisgros. I simply had no time to eat, and even when I could find a few minutes for myself, I was so utterly exhausted that, for the first time in my life, I didn't care about my meals. Anyone who has ever been in a similar situation knows that such a diet is foolproof, but hard to duplicate in ordinary life.

I think one day I will write the ultimate diet book, stringing all these diets into one megaprogram. It will consist of the Drinking Man's, Hot Fudge Sundae, Popcorn, and Bulk diets, along with others I declined along the way, like Beverly Hills, Stillman, Scarsdale, Bloomingdale's, and Atkins.

The rule will be to go from diet to diet, day after day. Every day you get to be on a different diet. If you gain weight, it's not your fault, you've been dieting.

Not all my diets were extreme. Periodically I would put myself on the right track and eat nutritious, fairly well-balanced meals, of fairly reasonable size, for weeks or even months. Then I would look and feel wonderful. But something always happened to mess me up.

My diets had no focus beyond losing pounds. I didn't understand cholesterol counts. I had heard vaguely about fiber, but I wasn't interested in learning any more. I exercised now and then, when I felt like playing baseball or football, but I didn't keep myself on a regular program of activity. I kept some sort of record of what I ate, but I wasn't sure how to use it. And most important, I didn't understand compulsion, even though I lived with it.

TOWARD A RATIONALE

These diets weren't a total loss because I learned something from each of them, either about diets or about myself. I was able to use what I learned in formulating my successful program for turning around my eating compulsion.

1 ALL OR NOTHING

Very early on, I learned that I couldn't expect myself to weigh and measure portions. To a compulsive person, eating is an all-or-nothing proposition, and any diet ignoring this is doomed to failure.

2 TRIGGERS

Monitoring my ups and downs on the diet seesaw taught me to recognize trigger foods, those few foods that are lethal to compulsive eaters—a personal Waterloo. (See chapter 4.) High-butterfat ice cream is my major trigger food. I can't stop at just one taste, and ice cream propels me into my worst bouts of overeating. Fried chicken is my second most powerful trigger. Even "healthy" fried chicken, breaded with oat bran and fried in unsaturated oil, can send me over the edge. Perhaps your triggers are different: chocolate, bread, salty foods?

3 SATIATION

As unsuccessful as the Popcorn Diet was for me, it introduced me to the concept of satiation. I now know that I can use popcorn as a fallback when I need to eat and to fill myself up, and as a "bridge food" that takes me from overeating to normal eating. I also learned, while dieting, how to eat something before my main meal, how to "eat dinner before eating dinner" (see chapter 8) so that I will not eat too much of the wrong foods later.

4 KEEPING A JOURNAL

A crucial strategy that evolved for me while I was hopping from diet to diet was keeping a record of everything I ate. I know now that I can use this record to learn when I eat and why, and I can use it as a tool to limit and control my eating (see chapter 8). You cannot kid yourself about "not eating much" if you see how much is written down.

5 LIFE CHANGE

Most important, it became clear to me that diets don't work. *I learned that only I could help myself; no one else could do it.* I had to stop and admit that I was living a self-defeating and unhealthy life-style, and then I had to take responsibility for change.

I couldn't follow a quick-fix program that had nothing to do with behavioral change. I couldn't take the easy road of fifteen pork chops or a hot fudge sundae for dinner. I really had to change my life, not just my menus.

In all my past diets I had gone through the motions of changing my behavior but I had no rationale for what I was doing. I was simply looking for a quick fix, an overnight weight loss. I didn't realize that changing my life-style went along with "dieting." I hadn't said: "I have a serious problem. I want to solve it. I intend to change my life for the better." Saying that and believing it were my essential first steps.

THE DIET SEESAW: A WOMAN'S POINT OF VIEW

"The specifics may be different, but David, you and I are very much alike," says an old friend who understands my addiction. Marianne is slim and elegant, but she started out as a fat child who was put on a diet at the age of seven. It was the first of many, many diets for her.

"I ate for comfort," she says. "Nowadays if a child is overweight you don't put her on a diet, you find out what is going on in her life. But through no fault of their own, my parents simply didn't know that important fact.

"As a child I moved with my family from our familiar New York home all the way to France. After my father died we all moved back to New York City. I really didn't know if I was a New York kid or a French girl. It took me quite a while to straighten out my identity and feel comfortable."

As she grew up, Marianne went up and down on the diet seesaw. She explained to me that women learn to measure themselves against society's standards for beauty rather than their own. They tend to become obsessed with these standards and finally internalize them. It seemed perfectly natural to struggle with her weight, Marianne pointed out, because "the women's side of this is: everybody is always on a diet." Her particular behavior—out-of-control eating—wasn't addressed because it fit in with the "I'm getting fat/ I have to diet before the swimsuit season" syndrome that occupies so many other women.

But Marianne found that she ate mindlessly, sometimes without even realizing that she was eating. And often her eating was triggered by anger. She believes that eating compulsively to suppress feelings of anger is very common in women.

Marianne was tough on herself. Whenever she binged, she followed her lapse with a strict diet.

"The only time in my life that I just gave up was when I was pregnant," Marianne admits. "I ate whatever I wanted to eat whenever I wanted to eat it. I made up for twenty years of dieting and I gained fifty pounds."

What turned Marianne around? It wasn't a death scare like my motivation. In fact, it was the exact opposite. She reached her fortieth birthday and was overwhelmed by the rich and varied opportunities of life. She made a *positive* leap into a new life-style.

Caring for her husband and children, Marianne faced daily temptations in the kitchen. But, like me, she was able to learn to enjoy preparing food for others and in that way to avoid eating it herself.

She found that she had a chunk of free time each afternoon, and she joined a nearby health club with a swimming pool. She discovered, to her delight, that she was an excellent swimmer, and she began swimming one mile every day.

This daily exercise became the cornerstone of a larger change in her life-style. From exercising, she moved to changing her eating habits. She has built her own system around her daily exercise, and each part depends upon the others. She still must guard against eating mindlessly while she prepares meals, and against eating out of anger.

"You have to accept the fact that compulsive eating is a problem that will be with you forever," she stresses. But if I swim my mile each day, I can stick to sensible eating."

DISMANTLING THE SEESAW

When you understand the nature of your compulsion, when you have a true motivation for change, and when you can put together a system of exercise and sensible eating, you can climb down from the diet seesaw. Take it apart and throw away the pieces—you won't need it anymore!

PART TWO

Your Road To Recovery

Chapter Four

Trigger Foods: Name Your Poison

Imagine that you are face to face with a platter of fried chicken, about to dive in.

You love food, sure, but that is not why you will eat it.

You may be hungry, but that is not why you will eat it, either.

You see that chicken and you are overcome by the need to control it, to conquer it, to have it all.

You can't take just one bite and then walk away. You can't eat just one four-ounce portion, skin removed. And once you have eaten all the chicken that is available, you cannot stop until you have consumed all the potatoes, all the bread and butter, and all the dessert on the table.

You are facing a trigger food.

A trigger food is any food that you cannot eat in moderation. You cannot take just one bite, just one spoonful, just one slice. I can eat one pretzel or one baked potato, but my universe does not allow for just one scoop of ice cream.

A trigger food is any food that sets off your cycle of compulsive eating. Stuffing yourself with a trigger food doesn't appease your hunger. Just the opposite—it will lead you to eat more food. You move on from fried chicken to ice cream to peanut butter, consuming everything available. You aren't hungry. Your body doesn't require any more nourishment. But once you have tasted your poison, you will continue to gorge yourself compulsively.

Triggers fall into four groups: fat, sugar, cholesterol, and salt. You can be sensitive to one or more of them. Fried chicken is a trigger for me, as are most foods containing fats. Candy, cake, ice cream, and any sugar except those occurring naturally in fruits also trigger my binges. Red meat, high in cholesterol, regularly sent me over the edge, straight into a binge. Only salt does not affect my eating patterns.

Some people are triggered by bread and butter. Some can't resist runny cheese. Some go nuts over coconut. Others are destroyed by salty potato chips.

Your trigger foods are the core of your addiction. They are your nicotine, your alcohol, and your heroin. Eliminate them and you will take a giant step toward controlling your compulsive overeating.

DETERMINE YOUR TRIGGER FOODS

Remember, triggers have a double effect: you overeat them, and you overeat other foods because of them.

If you are a compulsive eater you probably already know your trigger foods and can list them easily. You may be stuck at first, so try these five mind games.

Mind Game 1: Think about your childhood. When you came home from school, did you sit down at the kitchen table for a glass of milk and a piece of cake, perhaps sharing with your brother or sister? Or, like me, did you stand at the freezer or the refrigerator devouring an entire cake or a whole box of cookies and not leaving one crumb for anyone else—even your mother? If this story sounds all too familiar, cake is one of your trigger foods.

Trigger Foods: Name Your Poison

Mind Game 2: You don't have to think all the way back to your childhood to isolate your trigger foods. This is probably a painful question, but when was your last binge? Try to remember it in detail. Get a pencil and paper, sit down, and write everything you ate while you were out of control. Start with the last food and work your way backward until you reach the first. Bingo! That first bite was your trigger.

Mind Game 3: Have you been to a large party, wedding, or graduation lately? Imagine yourself at one of these events as cocktails are served. You know that soon the waiters will emerge from the kitchen carrying trays laden with hors d'oeuvres. There you are, closer than anyone else to that magic kitchen door. It opens and the waiters march out. Imagine each tray as it appears and passes before your appreciative face. Crudites? No thanks. Spareribs? Yes. Knishes? Yes. Fried shrimp? Yes, yes, yes. This is a veritable trigger gala.

Mind Game 4: Take a walk through your supermarket, without a cart. (I am not suggesting a gourmet shop, because trigger foods are usually accessible and affordable, since you eat them all the time.) Go up and down all the food aisles, at a brisk pace, and look at the products on both sides. Quickly note those foods you feel inclined to devour on the spot. Consider also the foods you could pick up and put down without so much as a nod. The temptations are likely to be your triggers.

One man I know was so overwhelmed by his trigger foods at the supermarket that he wore a sharp-edged ring when he shopped. He used it to slit open packages of potato chips. He could finish an entire bag before anyone noticed, and not even stop to put it in his cart.

Mind Game 5: Now ask yourself, "If this were my last day on earth, what would I eat?" (If you were not compulsive, you might consider what you would *do* during your final hours, and you would come up with some pretty creative answers. But if you are a CE, it is a given that you would eat.) The foods you choose to comfort your last moments on earth are likely to be those warm, fuzzy friends you have loved for years, your triggers.

By now you should have your list.

ELIMINATE YOUR TRIGGER FOODS

First, the bad news: You have to give up your trigger foods for the foreseeable future.

Now, the good news: You can take the future one day at a time, or even one meal at a time. Some people even clock themselves by the hour.

But you need a push—you need motivation to begin. In my case, it was the life-or-death cholesterol threat. I can't think of a stronger motivation, but there are other reasons for you to change. These reasons all come under the heading "Quality of Life." You want to look better, feel better, accomplish more.

Perhaps, like me, you graduated from buying clothes at the husky boys' shop to buying nothing-that-ever-looked-right at the fat men's shop. Again, like me, you may not think it's cute when your young children innocently announce: "You're fat!" Or maybe you cringe a little when your teenage daughter asks, "What size are those jeans you're wearing?"

Perhaps you are one of the 33 percent of American women who wear dress size fourteen or over. Shopping for clothes can be a nightmare because most of the really pretty clothes stop at twelve or fourteen. You are starting to fear that you will lose that special man, or that special job, to a slimmer, more attractive woman. And you know if that happens, you will just go on an eating binge to bury your sorrows and prove to yourself how worthless you really are.

How about some positive motivation? A newly married friend of mine looks forward to a blissful life—if only she can overcome her food addiction. Another friend remembers when her children thought she was as beautiful as a movie star. She knows she can be that way again. And Marianne, the woman I told you about in

Trigger Foods: Name Your Poison

chapter 3, was delighted to find that turning forty expanded her horizons.

Trigger foods don't help you to live longer, they don't help you to live better, and they don't help you to look better. Who needs them? They are your addictive substance, like cocaine or heroin is to a drug addict.

ELIMINATE YOUR TRIGGER FOODS: FIVE STEPS

Conquering your trigger foods requires pure common sense—the most important ingredient in my program.

1. Make a list of all your trigger foods and commit it to memory. Awareness of these foods should become as natural to you as breathing.

2. Get rid of all the trigger foods in your house. Don't plan to devour them over the weekend and then start this program Monday. Throw them out now! You are not harming or depriving yourself; you are making your life a little easier.

Apologize to the other people at home. If you live with someone who can take one spoonful of Haagen Dazs Deep Chocolate and then push away the dish, saying, "I'm just not hungry," he or she probably won't understand why you have to take this drastic step. Assure the people you love that they will have their treats available as soon as you become stronger, and that you definitely intend to become stronger.

It is a major victory when, after you have identified your triggers and thrown them out of the house, you can allow them to come back in again because you have learned to resist them. Reaching this point can entail a long process, and everyone's timetable is different, but the wonderful moment will arrive for you.

My children have ice cream and cookies in the house now, and it really doesn't bother me. But I never could have started this program if I had remained surrounded by temptation at home.

3. Don't hedge your bets. You cannot be selective about getting

rid of trigger foods. Don't hold on to one special favorite for auld lang syne. They all have to go.

The reason is obvious: trigger foods work in combination and they work alone. An ice-cream cone in one hand and a hot dog in the other may be lethal for you; if so, an ice-cream cone in each hand will be equally lethal.

If you dump four out of five foods on your list, that fifth will still do you in.

4. Remember that you can't sanitize a trigger food. Skinless breast of chicken dipped in egg white, rolled in oat bran, and fried in safflower oil is still fried chicken. If fried chicken is on your list (and it probably is), you cannot eat it.

Trigger foods have nothing to do with calorie counts, cholesterol levels, and balance. They are a nutritionist's nightmare because they just don't add up. Forget the charts and throw out the fried chicken.

5. Face the fact that eliminating trigger foods will be painful. But the pain will be short term. You will be delighted to find yourself getting stronger each time you say no.

IT REALLY WORKS

A newly married friend of mine asked me about trigger foods because she wanted an eating program that made sense for her. She quickly figured out which foods were dangerous, made her list, and memorized it. Then off she went to a dinner party. Here is her description of the evening.

"The hostess filled a table with killer hors d'oeuvres: salami, brie and crackers, caviar and cream cheese, fried chicken wings. I love this stuff! But I know that salt and fat do me in, and almost everything on that table was a trigger. So I smiled at my husband, nibbled on plain crackers, and drank some wine. I didn't feel deprived and no one noticed, because I was eating and drinking along with the other guests.

"When the main course was served, I realized I was in luck! It was a pasta primavera made with olive oil and no cream. I ate a reasonable amount and enjoyed it, and somehow I wasn't driven to overeat as I usually am. Then I had some salad, and finished the meal with fruit and coffee.

"Brownies were served too, and for a moment my eyes glazed over, but I declined. And by that point it wasn't so hard—I was feeling quite proud of myself.

"Naturally I weighed myself the next morning. Would you believe I actually lost two pounds? If I had started on those killer hors d'oeuvres I would have failed again and gained weight!"

WORST CASE

Okay, you isolated your trigger foods. You made your list, memorized it, and then mercilessly banished all triggers from your kitchen and your life. You were doing marvelously and then—who knows why—you fell. This is something every CE can recognize: out of the blue, for no apparent reason, something went wrong. One of your poisons sneaked up on you, you gave in, and you tumbled all the way back to square one. And there was nothing to break your fall.

I won't be condescending and say, "There, there, it doesn't matter." You are a grown-up, and you know what you did and where it landed you. Just remember how good you felt about yourself before you slipped! The sooner you pick up the pieces and get yourself back on the program, the sooner you will feel that way again. You can start again and you will be better off than you were the last time. You haven't lost all your will or self-knowledge. Don't make a big deal of your slip—just get back on track. Being back at square one simply means saying no again for the first time.

And just because you lost control, don't give up on the rest of your program. Don't stop exercising! Continue to write in your food journal! Doing these things will help you to regain self-control.

Your fall will be harmful only if you use it to get off this program for an extended time; that is, only if you give up.

A WORD ABOUT ICE CREAM

Ice cream seems to be a universal trigger food. It is sweet, creamy, and cold, and it slides right down with no effort on your part. No food could be easier to overeat.

And there are no "normal" portions. What constitutes a portion of ice cream—a spoonful, a scoop, a pint? For a compulsive eater, it is as much as he or she can lay hands on.

When I was eating compulsively, I had my ice-cream binges down to a science. I would buy three single-pint cartons from the grocery store, bring them home, and start eating immediately, even though the ice cream was rock hard.

I dug through the first pint with the help of a serrated spoon. Meanwhile, I had the second pint softening in my gas oven with the pilot light on. The third was doing a slow melt, too—I was sitting on it.

I managed to eat all three pints in sequence without missing a beat. By the time I had finished the first, the second had softened in the oven. And by the time I had consumed that one, the third was ready to eat. For years, I depended upon this system for my ice-cream fixes.

This is a self-portrait of a compulsive eater and his poison. I think a lot of other people can see themselves in the picture.

ERSATZ ICE CREAM

There are some acceptable substitute ice creams around that are low in sugar and cholesterol. American Glacé, Vitari, and nonfat frozen yogurt, among other desserts, can almost fool you into thinking that you are eating something sinfully rich. Should you eat them on this diet program?

In the beginning, no. After a month, if ice cream is a major trigger for you, still no. These desserts might propel you into a binge just like the real thing could do.

But once you are firmly into this program, you can give them a try. I don't mean that you should buy three pints and imitate my mother-hen routine. Instead, think of them as a fallback and put them in the same category as potato crisps and spicy popcorn.

When you want a treat, try one of these desserts. Can you stop at a small portion? Does eating it satisfy your urge for something cold and sweet? If you have answered "yes," then feel free to enjoy it. But if you find that the ersatz ice cream has awakened your urge to eat compulsively, throw it away and forget it!

For my friend Toni, diet ice cream acts as a trigger exactly as regular ice cream does. She will eat all she brought home in one sitting. Toni has decreed: no more ersatz ice cream.

Even if you can eat an ice-cream substitute, be careful—sometimes the shops selling these frozen desserts pack more calories than you expect into your cup. The culprit is something called overrun, the amount of air beaten into the dessert mix. When the overrun is less than the manufacturer recommends, you get more dessert and less air. Hence you get more calories.

You may also be getting more than the four ounces usually advertised as containing the caloric total. You think you are buying a four-ounce serving, but your friendly ice-cream purveyor may be serving you eight ounces—double the amount and therefore double the calories.

Ask for the number of ounces you want. Have the server weigh your portion. That is the only way to ensure that you are really getting a low-calorie treat.

ALCOHOL: THE TRIGGER'S TRIGGER

Jessica is a beautiful actress you may have seen on television game shows and sitcoms. She had been fighting a battle with her escalating weight, and she had come to prefer appearing on game shows. In these shows, the camera concentrated on her face and she was photographed sitting behind a desk.

She started my program wholeheartedly and has made excellent progress so far. She has helped me, too, with this important insight.

Jessica says: "My mother used to tell me not to drink because I might 'go too far' with a boy. The truth is that if I have wine with dinner, I will go too far with dinner! Just a little alcohol lowers my resolve, melts my willpower. If I have a drink, I head straight for my trigger foods, and from there it is disaster. Alcohol is a trigger for my triggers."

For many people, a drink is a push toward overeating. If Jessica sounds like you, skip that drink!

For me, having a drink or refusing it is usually a matter of whether I want to consume the extra calories. But there is one exception. Sometimes I sense that I am about to go over the edge, that I am having trouble resisting that cookie or that pastry. If I have a glass of wine instead of dessert, I feel that I have given myself a treat and I can forget the sweets. When you are in that weakened state where your two strongest options are a trigger or a glass of wine, the wine is preferable—if it is not a trigger for you, and if you do not have any problems with alcohol.

TRIGGER SITUATIONS

"I don't really have trigger foods as much as I have trigger situations," says Max, who works with food all day in his job as a corporate chef. The temptation to pick and taste is very strong for him, for me, and for anyone in the food business.

Max explains: "If I allow myself to pick at the foods I am preparing, I ignite a real trigger situation. I know I will continue eating for the rest of the day."

His trigger situations work in exactly the same way as trigger foods do: they cause overeating at the time and they lead to extended overeating for a longer time period.

Judy, a free-lance editor, finds that meeting a demanding deadline can be a trigger situation. As the clock ticks on, she fights the need to stuff her mouth with food—any food. Whatever she eats under this emotional stress can trigger a binge. If her real trigger foods were available, if she hadn't thrown them out, as I advised earlier in this chapter, the danger would be even greater.

A DEADLY COMBINATION

There are many possible trigger situations, and when they combine with trigger foods they can do enormous damage.

Roberta was getting her teenage daughter, Lisa, ready for a summer bike trip, and they were both tired and nervous. Lisa didn't know any of the other kids on the trip and she wondered if she was up to the physical challenge of biking several hundred miles. So she bombarded her mother with: "Where are you sending me? Why didn't you let me buy a better bike? You don't care about me? You are being so obnoxious!"—and the rest of the adolescent litany. Roberta felt unappreciated, exhausted, and angry. "Just one more word from this child," she told herself, "and I will have to eat ice cream. I can't help myself. I need some sweetness."

Ice cream was Roberta's main trigger, and the combination of her unhappy feelings and her trigger food promised to be devastating. Fortunately, Roberta had the good sense to take a step back. She went into the kitchen and made a huge batch of spicy popcorn for herself and her daughter. They forgot about packing for a while, and the trigger situation passed without harm.

Danny, a college junior, was talking to his professor about a poor exam grade. Danny pointed out that he had indeed answered the questions as the professor had required and that his essay had covered all necessary points and covered them well. "You're right," the teacher admitted. "I marked you too low. But you should have come in last week. All the grades are already in the computer. Sorry."

Danny fought the double urge to punch his teacher and then run out to the nearest fast-food shop.

It is extra hard to face these double whammies: not only are we in the middle of a trigger situation, a trigger food is close at hand and seems comforting and irresistible. Turning to fallback foods can really help at times like these. So can some of the other strategies you will find in chapter 8, such as projecting yourself sixty seconds into the future, talking to yourself, and going public with your diet.

COMMON SENSE

I keep coming back to that magic concept, common sense. First, I told you that you couldn't sanitize a trigger food. When you fry chicken, you end up with fried chicken, no two ways about it. But then I told you that you might be able to get around ice cream by eating other frozen desserts. How can that be?

Imitation ice cream may or may not act as a trigger for you once you are strongly committed to your diet. Only you can determine whether it will harm you, and only you can judge when you are ready to test it. Make the determination for yourself at the appropriate point.

For me, fried chicken is somehow more deadly than many of my other triggers. And I believe you will find that your major trigger or triggers can't be redeemed, either. Believe me, some things are better written off.

Others may become easier to handle. For instance, sugar-rich desserts no longer tempt me the way they once did; I can say no to cakes, cookies, and candy much more easily than I could before. I treat the entire category of dessert as a trigger, or trigger situation, and I go from my main course directly to my espresso or foaming cappucino. Dessert is simply not necessary.

I like to believe that I have eliminated sugar from my diet, yet I know that I still ingest it in the form of fructose when I eat fruit. Fructose and sucrose break down in your body in the same way, so that your body doesn't know whether you've eaten a brownie or a bunch of grapes. But I am not *psychologically* dependent on sugar.

Those extra calories I allow myself when I am in control will not do me in. Those calories I mindlessly gulp when I am out of control will trigger a binge.

I am not a doctor and I cannot give you medical reasons for the trigger phenomenon. I don't know if it is physical or psychological in nature—maybe it is a subtle combination of both.

I can't say that when you eliminate your trigger foods you will physically eliminate your need to overeat. You will have to be on guard most of the time and you will have to think consciously about resisting foods. (As a compulsive eater, you already spend most of your time thinking about food, so this is not a great leap.)

The trigger path to overeating may be the most persistent in your life, as well as the most destructive. But I can say with confidence that if you identify and conquer your triggers, you will see a real change in your patterns of living. You will feel great! And your strength will increase each time you say no.

Beating your trigger foods is not easy, but it is exhilarating!

Chapter Five

THE CHOLESTEROL CONNECTION

Until December 1987, food was killing me and I was doing very little to fight back. That food was loaded with cholesterol and saturated fats, so that my total blood cholesterol level was 324, and my weight hovered around 300, hitting an all-time high of 313.

I lived with stomachaches and nausea. I felt rotten most of the time and I suffered from chronic digestive problems brought about by compulsive eating. I knew that the worst of compulsive eaters ate until they felt they were about to explode. I was beginning to feel that I was the second worst: I ate and ate until I became nauseous, and I didn't stop even then.

But I was never a bulimic. I was so possessive of my food that I wouldn't give it up. I worked to get that food. I chewed it. I swallowed it. There was no way I was going to let it go, even if I was hunched up with nausea. A bulimic reasons: "I'll eat it and then I'll throw it up, so I didn't really eat it." That line of thought was not for me—I really ate it and I kept it.

I ate until I was in severe pain. I used to stay up all night, unable to sleep, taking medications that never worked. I had a vision of my stomach as being full of gas bubbles and when I swallowed the medicine I expected it to chug around and eat up all the bubbles—but the bubbles always won. I used to get pains so often that I thought I had ulcers. (When I controlled my wild eating the pains went away. Amazing how that works.)

When I overate I felt lethargic; I didn't want to move. I had to sit in a chair bent over, trying to make the nausea go away. Strange as it may sound to a normal person, I was so disgusted with myself for eating that I just kept on eating. Full of self-pity, I sank deeper and deeper into the pit.

My social plans centered around going to restaurants and eating as much as I could in public without embarrassing myself. When I went on trips to France, I packed clothing a size or two larger than I currently needed, because I expected a weight gain of two pounds a day. Through all this I had never given a thought to my cholesterol!

And I never would have gone to my doctor if I hadn't been bitten by a tick one winter day in the country. I guess I wasn't looking for a real way out of my problems at that time. I was still hoping for that quick fix or magic pill.

Fortunately I did see the doctor and he told me that I had no more time to fool myself, that unless I lowered both my weight and cholesterol I might soon be dead. When I heard him, and saw those alarming numbers, I finally had to admit how sick I really was.

I hadn't been ready to admit my sickness until the doctor's warning introduced the cholesterol factor. When he told me I wouldn't live to see my children grow up, I finally conceded that I was in trouble.

Then all the unconnected scraps of motivation I had been gathering and storing finally came together, galvanized by that shock, and I threw myself into the task of saving my life.

That December, I found myself in Toronto visiting a business connection. As I was leaving, he handed me a large baker's box of pastries to take home: croissants, danish, and other buttery baked goods. I accepted the parcel out of habit—when I got gifts of food I generally finished them down to the last crumb. Without thinking I carried the box to the airport and through customs. Then I stopped. I took that big box of pastries into a coffee shop and put it down on an empty table. I turned and walked away, leaving it there. It wasn't easy, but I kept on walking. I had made my decision.

I began my life-change program at the worst possible time for a compulsive eater—the Christmas season. (How many times have you been advised: "Don't start a diet during the holidays!"?) It would have been easy to say: "I'll throw out the ice cream and cake on January first," relying on the number-one crutch for a compulsive eater, procrastination. But I knew that I had to act immediately.

MY NEW LIFE

Zeroing in on my elevated cholesterol levels, I changed my diet and I began to exercise regularly. *I soon found that controlling my cholesterol meant controlling my weight.*

Doctors know that there is a strong connection between overweight and high cholesterol levels and they urge their patients to lose weight as a first step in lowering cholesterol. I found that the connection works both ways: I began my diet by lowering my cholesterol, and I learned that weight loss went along as a bonus.

Of course, cholesterol was not the only dragon I had to slay. Clearly, I had to conquer my compulsive eating habits in order to make any progress at all. There are many cholesterol-lowering diets around, but they often are hard for a compulsive eater to follow because they are extreme, rigid, or bland.

Until that tick bit me, I had been destroying myself as only a compulsive eater can, and then I began to reverse the process using the very energy that had fueled my eating compulsion. I read everything I could find about cholesterol. I put together my own program and I worked at it energetically. I knew I had to do this for myself. There would be no miracle cure.

SHOCK TREATMENTS

The key to any life change is your own internal decision. No amount of nagging, no amount of throwing yourself into Weight Watchers' programs and Diet Center clinics and Optifast programs is going to work without your own deep commitment. If it doesn't come from within, you are going to fail.

A serious scare can be the best thing for any kind of compulsive person. I have a friend who used to be an active alcoholic and is now a recovering alcoholic. He became very interested in beekeeping, put up several bee houses on his property, and started spending a lot of time with his bees. His wife was pleased that he had a hobby.

What he was doing was keeping his Scotch in the bee house. He knew no one would go in there and go through the thousands of bees to get to the Scotch. He had his life-changing scare when somehow he got too drunk out there in the bee house and he was badly, almost fatally, stung. That shock turned him around and saved his life.

Something similar happened to an attorney I know very well. We were walking down the street one day when he broke into a sweat and couldn't continue walking. It turned out that his arteries were clogged and he needed valve-replacement surgery. He was only in his forties, but he was in trouble with heart disease.

I was lucky; I didn't have the ultimate shock. I wasn't almost stung to death by bees and I didn't have to have my chest cut open and have my plumbing replaced or Roto-Rootered out. I was scared into change by two high numbers—my weight and my cholesterol. The cholesterol frightened me infinitely more than the weight ever had.

THE CHEMICAL VILLAIN

By now, everyone on the planet seems to know what cholesterol is: a fat-like, waxy substance produced by the body and also obtained through the diet, mainly from animal fats. When you eat foods rich in cholesterol or saturated fats, you can raise the level of cholesterol in your blood.

You can learn about cholesterol in detail from any of several fine books, among them: *Cholesterol: Your Guide for a Healthy Heart* by the editors of Consumer Guide, *Good Cholesterol, Bad Cholesterol* by Eli M. Roth, M.D. and Sandra L. Streicher, R.N., and *The 8-Week Cholesterol Cure* by Robert E. Kowalski. For our purposes, I will highlight a few facts.

HDL (high-density lipoprotein) cholesterol is considered the "good" cholesterol. It moves through the body to the liver, where it is excreted through the bile. LDL (low-density lipoprotein) cholesterol is "bad," because it is deposited along the artery walls, narrowing the channels through which blood flows to the heart. LDL cholesterol can block off coronary arteries and lead to a heart attack or stroke.

When you want to find out how your body is handling cholesterol it is a good idea to have a blood test. You then can expect to receive numerical results that indicate your total blood cholesterol level, your level of HDLs, and your LDL level.

Your blood cholesterol number reflects the milligrams of total blood cholesterol per deciliter of blood (mg/dl). When testing shows that your total blood cholesterol number is low and the HDLs are proportionately high, you—or your heredity—must be doing something right.

If you can lower your total cholesterol and LDL levels, you can decrease your chances of coronary heart disease.

HOW CAN YOU CHANGE YOUR NUMBERS?

If you are at high risk for heart disease (if your total cholesterol level measures 240 or above) or are borderline high risk (with a total cholesterol level of 200–239) you must bring your numbers down. Proper diet will be your first and most powerful weapon. *Two substances that do not belong in your diet are dietary cholesterol and saturated fats.*

Cholesterol occurs mainly in foods of animal origin, like beef, lamb, pork, veal, high-fat dairy products, and egg yolks. (See chapter 5 for a more complete list.) Obviously, when you eat foods that contain a lot of cholesterol, you can directly increase your own blood cholesterol.

Saturated fats are fats that are solid at room temperature. They are mainly of animal origin, but a few come from vegetable sources. Foods containing saturated fats are meats, milk, butter, cheese, lard, egg yolks, caviar, coconut oil, palm oil, and chocolate.

Human beings do not require any saturated fats in their diet! And eating these fats can raise your level of total blood cholesterol, just as ingesting cholesterol itself can.

OTHER FATS

All dietary fats are not created equal. Many foods contain fats that are polyunsaturated or monounsaturated.

Polyunsaturated fats are liquid at room temperature and are of vegetable origin. When you eat them *instead* of saturated fats, they can lower total cholesterol levels. Polyunsaturated fats are found in walnut, safflower, sunflower, corn, soybean, and sesame oils.

Monounsaturated fats, also liquid at room temperature, are found in olive oil, peanut oil, and canola oil. They decrease LDL cholesterol while they maintain or increase HDL cholesterol.

When you see a vegetable oil that is labeled *hydrogenated* or *partially hydrogenated,* you are looking at a normally unsaturated fat that has been chemically treated to become partly saturated. Why would anyone want to alter a perfectly good unsaturated fat? To make it last longer on the shelf and to make it resemble butter. Margarine contains partially hydrogenated oils but tub margarines contain less of these oils than stick margarines.

Remember that all fats, the unsaturated as well as the saturated, are high in calories. One gram of fat contains more than twice the calories of a gram of carbohydrate or protein. Using the recipes I provide in chapter 10, you will be able to cook with minimal amounts of oil. These recipes will help you to decrease the fat content of your diet.

When you cut out foods high in cholesterol and saturated fats and instead eat cholesterol-free foods like grains, fruits, and vegetables, and low-cholesterol poultry and fish, you have a fighting chance of lowering your cholesterol levels. Adding fiber to your diet gives you an even better chance.

FIBER

Fiber in your diet will help you to lower cholesterol and will promote good health in other ways as well.

Dietary fiber comes from plant cells—it is found in foods that grow. You can't digest it and your body can't absorb it, but you need it. There are two types of dietary fiber, insoluble and soluble.

Insoluble fiber cannot be dissolved in water. This is the kind you find in wheat bran, whole grains, and many vegetables. It is important to your regularity and it helps prevent intestinal diseases.

Soluble fiber can be dissolved in water. It is helpful to you because it interferes with the body's ability to absorb cholesterol and it also decreases cholesterol production by the liver. Yet, while it lowers total blood cholesterol and LDL levels, it does not lower the levels of "good" HDL. Oat bran is rich in soluble fiber, as are oats and many vegetables and fruits.

Both kinds of fiber belong in your daily diet and I include foods rich in both on my Yes list (see chapter 6). But in this program I particularly stress soluble fiber, because scientific research and my own experience have shown it to be very valuable in reducing cholesterol levels.

WHY OAT BRAN?

Oat bran contains a high proportion of soluble fiber and is easy to incorporate into your meals in the form of muffins and cookies, as well as cereal. Let me stop here to clear up a confusing point. One hundred grams of oat bran *contains* 14 grams of soluble fiber; it is not itself pure soluble fiber.

In Dr. James Anderson's important studies at the University of Kentucky, published in the early 1980s, subjects consumed oat bran daily as part of a low-fat and low-cholesterol diet and lowered their LDL cholesterol levels significantly. My total cholesterol level dropped from 324 to 175 in one year when I consumed 50 grams of oat bran a day in the form of muffins and cereals.

You can get soluble fiber from other sources than oat bran. Oatmeal, for example, contains about half as much soluble fiber as oat bran does and is very helpful in lowering cholesterol. Dried beans, black-eyed peas, green peas, sweet potatoes, broccoli, Brussels sprouts, corn, apples, oranges, grapefruit, and bananas all add soluble fiber to your diet. It is a good idea to include these legumes, vegetables, and fruits in your menus.

OAT BRAN COMPARED TO OTHER FOODS

In many cases, you would have to eat large portions of other foods to get the same amount of soluble fiber you can get from smaller amounts of oat bran.

You would have to eat 15.5 times as many apples as oat bran, by gram weight, for your fiber, 23.3 times as many oranges, 17.5 times as many bananas, and 46.6 times as many peaches. Among the vegetables, beans stand out as being very high in soluble fiber. But you would have to eat 4.2 times as many lima beans as oat bran, by gram weight, to get your fiber, or 3.7 times as many white beans.

How about other vegetables? By gram weight, you would need 7.7 times as much corn or 28 times as much asparagus to match oat bran's fiber content.

WHY MUFFINS?

The best news I discovered while I was working out this program is that three little muffins can fill your oat-bran quota. Made according to my recipe, each muffin contains 16 grams of oat bran, bringing your soluble fiber consumption up to 48 grams. That's a lot of asparagus.

Moreover, muffins made according to my recipe are only 78 calories apiece and contain no cholesterol. Each muffin has only 1 gram of fat and that fat occurs naturally in the oat bran itself.

I don't believe in making a sweet, fat-loaded, cakelike muffin and then pouring in the oat bran. The oat bran won't cancel out the calories and cholesterol. There is a 2- to 2½-ounce muffin being marketed that contains 255 calories, 12 grams of fat, and 60 milligrams of cholesterol. Another brand of muffin of the same size has 225 calories, 11 grams of fat, and 43 milligrams of cholesterol. Let the buyer beware.

RATE YOUR FOODS

If you have a cholesterol problem and a weight problem (I consider them in tandem because they are so closely connected for me), then every time you face a food you have to make a decision about whether you are going to eat it. This book will help you with your food decisions and will even help you come to make them automatically. First, it will give you information about the foods you can and cannot eat.

Read chapter 6 and refer to the Yes list and the No list. This is the simplest first step in the process of rating your foods. For example, the Yes list contains olive oil, so you know that if a recipe calls for this oil and no others, that recipe is acceptable at least as far as unsaturated fats are concerned.

The Yes list tells you that just about all the vegetables you can imagine are acceptable, and it mentions many specifically. If you are planning to eat vegetables, another decision is simplified. The Yes list tells you that fish is acceptable, and that poultry is, too.

Now stop a minute and think about your triggers. Think about calories, too, in a very general way. Suppose you are planning to eat that old standby, chicken. If you eat too much chicken breast, even grilled chicken breast, you can still consume too much cholesterol. If you were to fry that chicken, even in olive oil, you could also go overboard in terms of calories, compounding the problem. I don't have to remind you that moderation does not come naturally to a CE! So triggers and calories can influence your cholesterol as well as your weight.

With so much on your plate—literally—how can you decide anything? Don't give up! Sticking to this total program will help you. Once you have eliminated your triggers, stopped bingeing, and begun to monitor your meals and record them in your journal (see chapter 8 for more about your food journal), your decisions will become easier.

THE VARIABLES

In terms of cholesterol, your food decisions involve a number of variables, some of which are helpful and some of which are harmful. The helpful variables are:
- monounsaturated fats
- polyunsaturated fats
- insoluble fiber
- soluble fiber

The harmful ones are:
- cholesterol
- saturated fats
- hydrogenated oils

I don't count calories on this program. Calorie content often is a function of portion size and common sense. You don't need scales and charts to know when you are eating something highly caloric—either because it is an oversize chunk of something or because it is full of sugar and fat. Remember, if it looks fattening, it probably is.

Triggers are foods that don't let you stop at just one bite. (See chapter 4.) When you start eating a trigger food, you lose control. You eat all there is of that food, plus all there is of all the other foods you can find. While there are general categories of trigger substances, only you can identify your own individual triggers.

However, in terms of your weight and your compulsive eating habits, you should add these two variables to the list:
- calories
- triggers

To help you remember all these factors, here is a simple, informal checklist. The variables are listed down the center. On the left is the Present column—check here if the variable is a factor in the food you are considering—and on the right is the Absent column—check here if the variable does not appear significantly in the food. This is an overall approach, intended to give you a feel for the different kinds of foods you are eating without bogging you down in minutiae and high-tech statistics.

THE VARIABLES

PRESENT   ABSENT

monounsaturated fats
polyunsaturated fats
insoluble fiber
soluble fiber

cholesterol
saturated fats
hydrogenated oils

calories
triggers

It is easy to check off foods according to the variables on the chart; do it on paper or even in your head. You can easily rate all the ingredients in any recipe you want to prepare. For example, try rating the ingredients in my recipe for Baked Potato Skin with Grilled Turkey and Onions (see chapter 10.) Here are the ingredients for one serving:

1 baked potato
1 tablespoon olive oil
2 slices onion
1 large slice turkey breast fillet
salt and pepper to taste
¼ cup balsamic vinegar
2 tablespoons chopped chives

The Cholesterol Connection

Taking each ingredient in turn, simply note whether each variable that applies is either present or absent. These are general, overall decisions. You don't need tables and you don't need math. Don't bother with categories that don't apply. For example, fiber is not a major consideration when you are deciding whether to eat turkey breast fillet.

How would you rate the potato on this chart? Insoluble fiber is present (remember, it is not necessary to measure precisely). Cholesterol and saturated fat are absent. Calorie content is not a factor. *Is it a trigger?* Probably not.

The olive oil is easy; it is monounsaturated. Only one tablespoon is called for, so the calorie factor is absent. The onion is included only for flavoring, in a quantity too small to rate. The turkey breast is low in cholesterol, fat, and calories, so check the Absent side for these harmful ingredients. The salt and pepper don't have to be considered. Neither does the balsamic vinegar. The chives are present in an amount too small to bother about.

These individual ingredients probably are not triggers, but that call is up to you. All the variables check out, but look at the recipe as a whole and ask one last question. When everything is put together, does the dish become one of your triggers?

If the final answer is no, prepare the dish and enjoy it.

Just to give yourself some practice, here is another recipe—from another book—that you can rate according to the variables chart. It is for Green Peas "French style," and it serves six. The ingredients are:

3 pounds fresh green peas
6 lettuce leaves
12 small onions
½ cup butter
1½ teaspoons sugar
2 teaspoons salt

The peas contain soluble fiber and are low in calories; the lettuce and the onions are the same. But butter contains both cholesterol and unsaturated fat, and is high in calories as well. The sugar adds unneeded calories and, more important, is likely to be a trigger. Even the salt is overdone here, and perhaps there is enough to provide a trigger. Taken as a whole, with its hefty doses of butter, sugar, and salt, this recipe may be a trigger dish: it is not a good way to get your vegetables.

Now try a scallop recipe (again, from another book). It is Scallops Baked in Shells (Coquilles Saint-Jacques), and it serves four to six. The ingredients for preparing the scallops are:

2 cups white wine
2 pounds scallops
½ teaspoon salt
½ pound mushrooms
¼ cup minced onions
1 tablespoon minced parsley
3 tablespoons butter
2 tablespoons water
1 teaspoon lemon juice

The sauce calls for:

¼ cup melted butter
¼ cup flour
2 egg yolks
¼ cup heavy cream
⅓ cup bread crumbs

The wine and ½ teaspoon of salt are used for poaching the scallops; they are discarded and they don't have to be rated. For the scallops, cholesterol is absent as a factor, as are saturated fats, and calories are low. The mushrooms, onion, and parsley together provide a little insoluble fiber and not much in the way of calories. The 3 tablespoons of butter are marked Present for saturated fats and cholesterol. Forget about the small amounts of water and lemon juice. The second part of the recipe requires ¼ cup of butter, again scoring Present for saturated fats and cholesterol. The butter in both parts of this recipe also adds a lot of calories. The flour adds nothing much in terms of fiber but it does give you some unwanted calories. Two egg yolks are loaded with cholesterol as well as calories. Saturated fats and cholesterol are definitely present in the heavy cream. If you make your own bread crumbs, then you can make sure that the bread doesn't contain saturated fats and cholesterol; if you use someone else's, fat and cholesterol can be either present or absent. Taken as a whole, this is a high-calorie recipe and may also be a trigger dish. You can do better by your scallops.

Perhaps this recipe is too easy too criticize, containing as it does the obvious villains, butter, cream, and egg yolks. But it is a good example of the kinds of dishes that people turn to when they want something elegant for a party. When you read my recipes in chapter 10, you will see that there is absolutely no reason to cook greasy, heavy, cholesterol-filled foods! The healthful dishes I give you are far more elegant and delicious.

EXERCISE, CHOLESTEROL, AND WEIGHT LOSS

Regular aerobic exercise will help you to improve your cholesterol numbers. It can lower LDL levels and raise HDL levels. It can also help speed weight loss because it burns up calories, both while you are exercising and for some time after you have finished. See chapter 7 for the full story on exercise.

Weight is more than a cosmetic consideration, since obesity can raise levels of blood cholesterol. Remember that losing weight is strongly connected with lowering cholesterol: each process will help the other to succeed.

Chapter Six

DAVID'S DELICIOUS FOOD PROGRAM

Recently I eavesdropped on three overweight gentlemen who were dining at my New York restaurant. I couldn't resist, because they were talking about dieting and talking about me.

They had heard about my weight loss and they were dubious. Undoubtedly I was on pills, said one. I had to be fasting, insisted another. I was taking Balkan sheep-fetus miracle shots, thought the third. They couldn't accept the real story because it seemed too simple and too good to be true. But it is true, and it is simply this.

I AM NOT ON A DIET

I have stopped eating a number of foods that are harmful to me, I have started eating other, more healthful foods, and I eat infinitely less than I used to. I don't take any medication, I don't use any gimmicks, and as far as these three guys are concerned, *I am not on a diet*.

Being on a diet means counting calories and measuring portions. It means feeling deprived. More important, "being on" implies eventually "going off" a diet. If you lose when you are on, you gain when you go off—the infamous yo-yo syndrome.

I changed my behavior in response to a threat to my health and my life. Instead of bingeing on fried chicken and ice cream, as I did for years, I now exercise daily, watch my cholesterol, and record in a diary everything that I eat.

Lowering cholesterol is the cornerstone of my program. It is central to my total life change, a change that involves brand-new patterns of eating, exercising, and thinking.

This book introduces you to my program of cholesterol reduction and weight loss and gives you the tools and the skills you need to follow it. If you follow this program, you will soon start looking and feeling better. If you do what I do, you will lose weight.

What can I call this program of cholesterol reduction, dietary change, behavioral change, and physical improvement? The world calls it a diet, so, using the general shorthand, I sometimes will refer to it as a diet, too. But every time you read "diet," please think: "a program for saving my life!"

Remember, I am only using a convenient term: this is not a diet in the usual sense of the word.

HOW TO USE THIS BOOK

I hope this isn't the first chapter you read. I know the temptation in a book of this sort is to flip through until you reach the heart of the book, the "diet." But this book is all heart—it tells you a lot more than what to eat and what not to eat. It tells you what compulsive eating has meant in my life and what it probably means in yours. It tells you about the value of exercise and the importance of keeping a food diary. It explains trigger foods and their importance to your weight-loss program. It gives you strategies that will help keep you on the program. Please don't take the "diet" out of context.

Before you put this life-change program together for yourself, it is important that you understand the philosophy it is based on. Every chapter tells you, in as many ways as possible, that my program depends upon common sense and taking responsibility for yourself. There are no gimmicks and no quick fixes. There are very few rules to follow. And most of my strategies and suggestions are subject to your own knowledge of yourself and your own good judgment.

For instance, many diets require that you eat portions of a specific size. This program doesn't. It is up to you to determine your own portion size. You will lose weight by cutting out foods that are high in cholesterol and saturated fats, rather than by controlling portions. Since every gram of fat has more than twice the calories of a gram of carbohydrate or protein, cutting fats out of your diet automatically reduces your calorie comsumption to some degree. Eventually, you will stabilize your own portion sizes as well because you will eat what fills you up at the time, and no more. A portion of chicken for me used to be a whole chicken. Now it is usually a quarter of a chicken, *and I don't have to think about it!*

Standard cholesterol-lowering diets allow you to eat some lean red meat, veal, and pork, since these meats can contain about as much cholesterol as chicken. My program says no to red meat because I have found it to be a trigger food for many compulsive eaters. For me, and for many other CEs, it leads to excess. So you will find red meats on my No list.

But remember, you will personalize this diet according to your own triggers. If you determine that beef, veal, and pork are not your poisons, then common sense dictates that you move them to your approved list.

The food lists I give you are nutritionally sound, even though they are not the strict constructions of doctors or nutritionists. The lists have worked for me. How many strict diets have worked for you so far? And if you were able to lose weight on those diets, how many times did you gain it all back?

Your most effective weapon will be your knowledge of trigger foods, those foods that bring on your binges. You will be better able to fight compulsive eating when you become aware of your trigger foods and eliminate them. (See chapter 4.)

Very possibly this fight may be a lifelong one, but it is hard to contemplate "forever." Think about eliminating trigger foods completely for twenty-four hours at a time. Maybe some day in the future the new, stronger you will be able to live with moderation. But for now, your addiction to food is as strong as an alcoholic's addiction to liquor. *Don't underestimate the power of your triggers.*

A WORD ABOUT BALANCE

When I was in high school, I used to go to football practice and listen to the coach as he carefully outlined what we were all supposed to do throughout the season. He would tell us that if we did a, b, and c, we would all be great players. In truth, a, b, and c often didn't add up. There are very few great football players.

Perhaps in the past you tried to regulate your diet according to the a, b, and c you learned from nutritionists. You studied food groups and calories and tried to put together low-calorie, balanced meals that would nourish you and reduce your weight.

But this balance theory didn't work. I know the reason, and you probably do, too. As a compulsive eater, you live in an all-or-nothing world. You can't stick to any program that requires you to weigh two ounces of this and three ounces of that. You know that these numbers are logical, but if they added up for you, you wouldn't be where you are today.

Nothing turns off a veteran dieter (even a non-CE) quicker than seeing a menu that measures food: 4 ounces tuna, ½ cup string beans . . . when people see that, they put down the book.

I am not asking you to diet by the numbers. I give you a list of foods approved by medical authorities for a low-fat, low-cholesterol eating program. There are no food supplements or gerbil foods. I give you delicious, easy-to-prepare recipes that I have developed and tested, based upon these approved foods. I do not tell you how much you can eat.

I also give you a list of foods to avoid, the No list, because these foods are high in saturated fats, cholesterol, and sugar. This list probably contains some of your old favorites. Face the fact that you can live without these killer foods. If you don't want to face that for the foreseeable future, try doing it one day at a time.

This is my personal program. It works for me and I want to share it with you. I expect you to tailor parts of it to suit your life. Only you can do this, because only you know your own limits and, even more important, only you know your own triggers.

HOW DID YOU GET HERE?

If you are a compulsive eater, you may have picked up this book because you felt desperate. Your eating problems have been around for a long time. When you were little, you learned that food often meant love and approval. "Here's a cookie for being so good," Mom would say, or maybe she would promise to bake a special chocolate cake if you got a good report card. And Grandma proudly bragged: "That child is such a good eater!"

As a kid, you probably started bingeing on junk food and then began out-of-control eating. Perhaps you were nagged about it by a parent or your peers, and you felt guilty and unattractive. Maybe you assumed that your "baby fat" would go away one day, but *mañana* never came.

Perhaps you learned early that if you didn't finish all the cake or all the ice cream after dinner, whatever remained would be gone by morning. You carried that lesson into adulthood, and now you can't stop eating the ice cream until it is all gone. There is a little kid still living inside you, sure that someone is going to steal your food the minute you turn your back.

Out on your own, in college or on the job, you just couldn't get away from temptation. Did you mysteriously gain weight when you left school and stopped playing sports? Luciano Pavarotti, the great tenor, was a soccer player of normal weight until he gave up sports to pursue his singing career. He just kept eating like an athlete in training.

Did your weight gain begin with domesticity? Once you married and started regular (and delicious) meals at home, did you find the pounds added up?

David's Delicious Food Program

But good meals weren't the whole problem. You didn't just eat, you binged; you didn't know when to stop. You ate until the refrigerator was empty and you felt as if you were bursting. Eating brought stress, and resisting food brought even more stress.

You tried diet after diet, but you were never able to control your addiction to food. You lost ten, twenty, thirty pounds and more, and gained it all back—more than once. And of course, you blamed the food, or your metabolism, or your hungry fat cells. You were awash in denial. Or you felt like a total failure.

Now you spend a lot of time and energy on food. If you're not eating, you're thinking about it and planning how and when to eat it. If you are the way I was, you calculate the time it takes for your spouse to go upstairs and come back down, so you can plan your secret dashes to the corner store for candy bars. When your boss compliments you on a job well done, you probably think, "Yes, this is a great contract. Where can I get some ice cream?"

You look forward to food shopping but you only stock up for one day at a time, because you know that when you get home, you will eat everything you bought. When I was eating compulsively, a cake never spent the night at my house.

You have a problem and you know it. Out-of-control eating has damaged your life and your health.

Solving this problem will require hard work. I can give you recipes and strategies that will help. I can tell you stories about my own life that you can relate to. I can explain how I turned my compulsion around. But I can't offer you a quick-fix diet or a magic pill. You bought this book for help—now you and only you must take over. The responsibility to change is yours alone. You have to scale that wall. This book is about reality, not about gimmicks.

Changing your life patterns for the better is a process, and you will face some painful moments. But I assure you that the pain will be short term, because as this diet takes hold you will get stronger and stronger. The payoff is that when you wake up in the morning, you won't be as fat as you were the day before.

For years, I was not willing to change my eating habits. Then I received the news that my health and my life were in grave danger because of these habits. That shock catapulted me into change.

You may not be facing danger—perhaps you are just facing your high-school reunion, or a closet filled with lots of stylish clothes that you can no longer wear. Are you ready for change?

CLEANING HOUSE: YOUR MIND

There is a very simple way to describe your food addiction: the cholesterol and the pounds are in your body, but the problem begins in your head. And that is where the solution begins—in your head.

The first step to that solution is confronting the fact that you are a compulsive eater. Be honest with yourself. Discard your rationalizations for the way you eat. Compulsive eating is a sickness.

How can you know if you are a CE? There is a one-second test. Answer this question: "Do I eat when I am not hungry?"

If the answer is yes, you are a CE. You can take your diagnosis further with this question: "Do I continue to eat when I am full, even when I feel stuffed?"

If you answered yes to that one, you have a bad case. You don't need complicated interviews or charts to tell you that fact. *But you are not alone. Many others are in the same situation.*

It is not enough to admit you are in the grip of a sickness. Now you must decide to do something about it. Many CEs admit their compulsion but go no further. They say, as I did for years, "Yes, I eat compulsively, but I can stop it any time I want to."

They say: "I've eaten all I want. I'm full and content. But I have to finish what's on the plate, on the table, and in the pot."

Or they say: "This is the last binge. I will just get this one out of my system and then I will never binge again."

It is time to wake up and tell yourself: "I've had enough of this! I don't want to kill myself with food! I want a normal life, starting now. I want a program I can stick to."

Read my anecdotes about my own battle with compulsive

eating. I know what it feels like to be out of control. I did something about it and you can, too.

CLEANING HOUSE: YOUR KITCHEN

Preparation for this diet is like spring cleaning, but more fun.

First, read the list of all the foods that you must eliminate. Add to that list your personal triggers, as you have determined them after reading chapter 4. Then, clean out your freezer, your refrigerator, and your pantry. Get rid of all those foods.

Don't get rid of them by eating them! A CE will try to wiggle out of taking responsibility by saying: "I'll just finish all this and then I'll start my diet on Monday." I know you've heard that one before.

Give the food away, but if there are no takers, throw it away. Yes, throw it in the garbage can, even though people on this planet are starving. Afraid of your guilt? It's time to feel a little guilty about stuffing your body with every piece of food you can find, about treating *yourself* like a garbage can.

Don't feel sorry for yourself! If you feel sorry for yourself you will overeat again.

I remember taking some Haagen Dazs and throwing it down the incinerator chute. I felt a deep sense of loss, and I asked myself dramatically: "What have I done?" Then I realized I hadn't done much. The pain passed quickly, and I felt great.

If you can throw away chocolate ice cream, you are on your way to recovery!

While you are dumping, think of all the wonderful meals you will soon be enjoying—meals free of foods that load your body with cholesterol and calories. Think of Grilled Swordfish on Melted Leeks, Roasted Mushrooms and Garlic Chez Louis, White-Clam Pizza, Linguine with Garlic and Anchovies. Keep dumping!

Your family will understand. Before long they will be able to keep ice-cream bars in the freezer again, because before long, you will be much better able to resist temptation. Once you have made some progress in this program, you will enjoy seeing them enjoy their treats. Not only that, you will happily pass out the ice cream to everyone else. (See chapter 8 for my strategy, "Feed Others Instead of Yourself.") For now, they can go out for ice cream without you.

CUISINE

Look at the Yes list of foods you can eat and enjoy. Then turn to chapter 10 and skim through my recipes. Which dishes particularly appeal to you? Read them more carefully, savoring them. Which one would you like to have for dinner tonight, and for lunch tomorrow? Which recipe seems the most appealing of all? Plan to reward yourself with that one at the end of the week.

Make a shopping list and then buy all the ingredients you will need for these recipes. Include food from the Yes list in this chapter and from the "Staples" list in chapter 10. You don't have to shop one day at a time for your food, as you did when your eating was out of control. These foods can spend the night in your pantry and your refrigerator.

Read chapter 10 to see what kitchen equipment you may need.

Look forward to eating some great meals. Using the food lists and recipes I give you, you will feed yourself very well. Most important, you will be able to limit fats and cholesterol without feeling deprived.

My list of approved foods is far from spartan. For instance, I think lobster is an excellent diet food because it is labor-intensive—you have to work hard to get the lobster out of the shell. I also recommend shrimp, mussels, salmon, grouper, swordfish, bass, skate, squab, and chicken, as well as oat bran, and wehani rice, and quinoa—grains that are available in supermarkets and specialty stores.

We all have to face difficult food decisions again and again, as we choose the healthful foods and resist the harmful ones. By using a basic core of low-cholesterol, low-fat, high-fiber foods, I simplify

David's Delicious Food Program

your daily (perhaps hourly) decision process. I concentrate on a few cornerstone recipes that are uncomplicated and fun to prepare.

The foods on my Yes list are considered prudent, but they are not dull. I am a chef and my interest in fine food borders on the obsessive. There is no way I would put together dishes that were uninteresting or even ordinary. I worked out all the recipes in this book for myself and tested them to my own satisfaction before including them. I have been serving some of them to diners at my New York restaurant, Chez Louis, and they have gotten raves. Changing your behavior does not mean giving up your enjoyment of good food.

START NOW!

Don't plan to start this diet next Monday. Start on Friday, and better yet, start with lunch on Friday. That will give a real boost to your willpower.

I know so many CEs who overeat wildly until Sunday at midnight, and then begin their diets at 12:01 Monday. In my New York City neighborhood I see food addicts prowling for those last pints of ice cream between 11:00 P.M. and 12:00 A.M. Sunday night. I know how they feel—I was one of them.

Sure, if you start Friday, you will have to face the weekend. But you will always have to face a weekend. And you will have to face a graduation, a wedding, a bar mitzvah. So what? All you can do is save your life.

THE FOOD LISTS

Here are my personal lists. I begin with nutritionally sound, medically approved foods, and then I add and subtract according to the trigger theory. You will personalize these lists by eliminating your own trigger foods and perhaps even by allowing yourself to eat some of mine.

For instance, I love chicken skin—that aromatic, crunchy, crisp-textured stuff that holds the chicken together. Amazingly, when I leave the skin on the chicken I prepare, my cholesterol doesn't rise and I don't gain weight. Moreover, I am not tempted to overeat chicken or anything else. So I allow myself to eat crunchy chicken skin. I don't eat it every day and I am careful to broil or roast chicken, and *never, never to fry it*. Chicken skin is not on my No list. Remember what you read in the trigger chapter (chapter 4) and ask yourself if it should be on yours.

You will be able to stay on this program because you can construct it so that it makes sense for you.

ABOUT THE YES LIST

This list is potentially vast, so you don't have to feel deprived.

I love juicy red grapes and those small, lusciously sweet Israeli melons—they are fun to eat and hunger appeasing.

I love potatoes, whether baked or served steaming, seasoned with flavorful salsa, or thinly sliced, highly spiced, and baked until crisp. My famous Chez Louis Potato Pie can serve six people and I use only four tablespoons of olive oil in its preparation. And my Killer Potatoes with Hot Chilies are not for the timid.

I like to use sweet, oniony leeks in my recipes. When they are "melted" or burnt they add a special dimension to the foods they flavor.

There are hundreds of fruits and vegetables available and acceptable—my list just skims the surface. You can eat grapes, apples, oranges, potatoes, leeks; in fact just about everything. I include the ones I commonly eat and invite you to add your own favorites.

The same is true for fish and shellfish. I list just the most common varieties, but please try all the tempting fish that is available. If you can't find some of the types of fish on my list—perhaps skate or grouper aren't always in your market—simply substitute the best and freshest fish that is offered. And forget the shellfish myth. Those heavenly lobsters, shrimp, clams, and oysters are not loaded with dangerous cholesterol, as we once believed. Not only are they low in the harmful kind of cholesterol, they contain

David's Delicious Food Program

noncholesterol sterols that scientists say may inhibit our absorption of cholesterol. They are very low in fat, as well.

Chicken, poussin (also known as "baby chicken"), and small game birds are excellent fare when grilled with just a touch of olive oil. And they keep you busy and satisfied while you enjoy them. I don't ask you to remove the skin from your poultry (except from duck), but if chicken skin triggers your binges, stay away from it. As I told you, chicken skin is not a trigger for me as long as the chicken is grilled or roasted. Determine for yourself whether it is a trigger for you. Although you must watch your consumption of animal fats, including fats in dairy products (they are all saturated, and therefore artery damaging), you can include unsaturated vegetable fats. Just be aware that all fats are high in calories, and use them sparingly.

You will enjoy, as I do, oat-bran muffins sweetened with sugar-free fruit preserves. Whole-wheat, sourdough pretzels made without fat or sugar are a crunchy treat available in many stores. Popcorn, hot and spiced, can be a bridge food, one that carries you from your state of overeating or food craving to a happier state of satiation. Nuts contain monounsaturated and polyunsaturated oils, and they are on the Yes list in terms of cholesterol. But they are high in calories, and I don't advise making a meal of them, or even a hefty snack. If they are your triggers (see chapter 4), give them up altogether.

You can drink wine with dinner or lunch if you choose, unless it is a trigger for you in some way (see chapter 4). But decide whether you can afford the non-nutritive calories that alcohol provides. Fruit juices may provide unwanted calories too, despite their nutritive value, so you won't want to overdo them. But I find that sugarless carbonated drinks are good choices, because they help to fill you up.

THE YES LIST

FRUITS

- APPLES
- APRICOTS
- BANANAS
- BLACKBERRIES
- BLUEBERRIES
- CANTALOUPE
- CRANBERRIES
- GRAPEFRUIT
- GRAPES
- HONEYDEW MELON
- ISRAELI MELON
- KIWIS
- LEMONS
- LIMES
- ORANGES
- PEACHES
- PEARS
- PINEAPPLE
- PLUMS
- RASPBERRIES
- STRAWBERRIES
- TANGERINES

VEGETABLES AND LEGUMES

- ARTICHOKES
- ASPARAGUS
- BLACK BEANS
- BEETS
- BOK CHOY (CHINESE CABBAGE)
- BROCCOLI
- BRUSSELS SPROUTS
- CABBAGE
- CARROTS
- CAULIFLOWER
- CELERY
- CHILI PEPPERS
- CORN
- CUCUMBERS
- EGGPLANT
- FAVA BEANS
- FENNEL
- GARLIC
- GREEN BEANS
- LEEKS
- LETTUCE
- LIMA BEANS
- MUSHROOMS
- NAVY BEANS
- OLIVES
- ONIONS
- PEAS
- PINTO BEANS
- PEPPERS (GREEN, RED, YELLOW)
- POTATOES
- SHALLOTS
- SNOW PEAS

David's Delicious Food Program

SPINACH
SQUASH, SUMMER AND
   WINTER
SWEET POTATOES
SWISS CHARD
TOMATOES
TURNIPS
ZUCCHINI

DAIRY
FROMAGE BLANC
NON-FAT COTTAGE CHEESE
NON-FAT PLAIN YOGURT
SKIM MILK

FISH
BASS
BLUEFISH
CATFISH
COD
FLOUNDER
HADDOCK
HALIBUT
PIKE
SALMON
SHAD
SKATE
SNAPPER
SOLE
SWORDFISH
TROUT
TURBOT
TUNA
WHITEFISH

SHELLFISH
CLAMS
CRAB
LOBSTER
MUSSELS
OYSTERS
SCALLOPS
SHRIMP
SQUID (CALAMARI)

POULTRY
CHICKEN
CORNISH HEN
DUCK (LEAN BREAST MEAT
   ONLY, NO SKIN)

POUSSIN (BABY CHICKEN) SQUAB
QUAIL TURKEY

FATS AND OILS
CANOLA
CORN SESAME
OLIVE SOYBEAN
PEANUT SUNFLOWER
SAFFLOWER WALNUT

SNACKS AND FALLBACKS
LENTILS SESAME SEEDS
NUTS SOYBEANS
POPCORN SUNFLOWER SEEDS
POTATO CRISPS
PRETZELS (FAT-FREE,
   SUGARLESS, WHOLE WHEAT)

DRINKS
CARBONATED WATER TEA
COFFEE WATER
DIET SODA WINE
FRUIT JUICES

HOW IT ALL STARTED: ABOUT FIBER

When I got the bad news about my soaring cholesterol count, I started eating a bowl of oat-bran cereal every morning. I had read the studies citing oat bran as an excellent source of soluble dietary fiber, which is useful in lowering cholesterol.

I bought sugar-free oat-bran flakes at a local health food store, but I found this cereal less than appetizing and a real bore. As I said earlier, it seemed to turn to cement in the bowl within thirty seconds of hitting the milk. And I didn't enjoy those few seconds of eating time, anyway. I desperately needed another way to get oat bran into my system, so I developed a delicious version of oat-bran muffins. Soon after that, I developed the recipe for my chewy oat-bran cookies. (The recipes are given in chapter 10.) Now I eat both muffins almost every day, either for breakfast or as a snack.

But oat bran is only part of a sensible eating program. It is not a miracle food, and it can't lower your cholesterol all by itself. You will not benefit if you eat oat-bran muffins for breakfast and fried chicken for lunch.

Insoluble fiber, such as that contained in wheat bran, is important to your health too, and whole-grain cereals and breads are a delicious part of my program. I have discovered seven-grain bread, a chewy loaf that is filling and fun to eat. I don't recommend specific brands of bread that you can buy in your supermarket because many breads from commercial bakeries contain sweeteners like corn syrup and honey. The breads I prefer come from my local bakery. If you stick with the supermarket, you should read bread labels carefully and find a brand that fits into this program and contains no trigger ingredients.

Texture adds another dimension to the enjoyment of food and that is one reason I like grains. Look for wehani rice, a chewy variety of reddish-brown rice with a nutlike flavor, and for several other new rice varieties on the supermarket shelves. Regular brown rice is good, too. Serve quinoa (pronounced *keen-wa*) as an alternative to rice. It is a Peruvian high-altitude grain that has a high protein content and an unusual flavor.

FIBER SOURCES: GRAINS, SEEDS, DRIED PEAS, AND BEANS

BARLEY	DRIED PEAS
BROWN RICE	LENTILS
CHICK PEAS	OAT BRAN
DRIED BEANS	OATS

QUINOA	FLATBREAD
SESAME SEEDS	OAT-BRAN MUFFINS
WEHANI RICE	OAT-BRAN COOKIES
WHEAT	PASTA (NON-EGG)
WHEAT BERRIES	PITA BREAD
WHITE RICE	SEVEN-GRAIN BREAD
WHOLE-GRAIN CEREALS	WHOLE-WHEAT BREAD

Some other foods containing soluble fiber are carrots, peas, corn, sweet potatoes, cauliflower, zucchini, apples, pears, grapes, and citrus fruits.

ABOUT THE NO LIST

These are the foods that contain saturated fats, cholesterol, and sugar. With a few exceptions, they are animal rather than vegetable products: meats, egg yolks, and high-fat milk products. But the No list also contains some saturated vegetable oils. (Saturated and unsaturated fats are discussed in chapter 5.)

If you can't face abandoning these foods forever, think about one day at a time. Twenty-four hours without lard is not so long!

Remember to personalize this food program. There is a gray area where some foods divide into trigger foods and into non-trigger foods, and that is where you have to tailor the lists to meet your own requirements. Veal is a perfect example of a gray-area food. In cholesterol content, it is not much different from chicken. If veal is not a trigger for you, then it is fine for you to eat lean veal, perhaps a paillard of veal. You may even be able to eat lean beef occasionally. But if you cannot eat beef sensibly, if one hamburger leads to five hamburgers plus French fries, then beef is a vicious trigger food that will take you way over the line both on calories and on cholesterol.

David's Delicious Food Program

THE NO LIST

BEEF
CAVIAR
HIGH-FAT, HIGH-SALT, LUNCHEON MEATS: HAM, PASTRAMI, CORNED BEEF, SALAMI, LIVERWURST, LUNCHEON ROLL, BOLOGNA, FRANKFURTERS, AND SO ON
LAMB
ORGAN MEATS
PORK AND PORK PRODUCTS
VEAL

BUTTER
CAKES, COOKIES, AND PASTRIES
CHOCOLATE
COCONUT
COCONUT OIL
CREAM
EGG YOLKS
HIGH-FAT CHEESES: TRIPLE CREAMS, BRIE, BLEU, STILTON, FORME, MOZZARELLA, CHEDDAR, AND SO ON
HYDROGENATED SHORTENING
ICE CREAM
LARD
MILK OTHER THAN SKIM
PALM OIL
SOUR CREAM

THE NUTS AND BOLTS: HOW TO PUT IT ALL TOGETHER

This program does not mandate your menus or restrict you to one from Column A and one from Column B. I'm a compulsive person just like you, and I won't insult your intelligence by pretending that someone else's logic works for people like us. *Choose your own foods for each meal, just as you choose your own portions.*

You may feel a little strange during the first few days, so let me walk you through the program.

BREAKFAST

The first few mornings you may not want to eat. Compulsive eaters often wake up feeling logy and full because they have snacked or binged late into the night. And the same compulsion that drives them to eat crazy amounts of food at night makes them starve themselves in the morning.

On my program you will change this pattern! You will eliminate your after-dinner binges and enjoy waking up full of energy. Train yourself to eat a morning meal. It is important for you to stabilize breakfast; if you skip this meal you will be tempted to make it up with interest later in the day—and night. Remember to record breakfast in your food diary (see chapter 8).

Your breakfast will not change from day to day, except as you choose to vary the cereal and fruit. Look for cereals that are fat free, high in fiber, and relatively low in sugar. Among the good ones are oatmeal, Wheatena, Shredded Wheat, Cheerios, Quaker Oat Bran, the Health Valley oat cereals, Grape Nuts, and Special K. I've seen good results with Total, even though it contains sugar.

I give you the option of fruit or juice in this breakfast, although I never drink juice myself. I have learned that fresh orange juice is one of my triggers: it makes me crave bacon and eggs and everything else on the breakfast or brunch menu. Many other people feel that a glass of juice offers too many calories too fast—all that fruit sugar just slides down. If fruit juice is not a trigger for you, then make a decision about whether you will drink it or whether you prefer to stretch out those calories by eating a cut-up orange or other fruit.

DAVID'S BREAKFAST
OAT-BRAN MUFFINS, MY RECIPE ONLY, AND/OR
HIGH-FIBER CEREAL WITH SKIM MILK
FRESH FRUIT OR JUICE
COFFEE OR TEA WITH SKIM MILK, IF DESIRED

LUNCH

Make sure you control your lunch environment whenever possible—one way to do this is to prepare your own lunch. If you buy lunch and take it to work, you may want to shop at a salad bar. When you eat out, stick to those restaurants you can rely on for the lean, healthful foods you will enjoy eating on this program. (Chapter 9 will help you.) Don't buy lunch or snacks from street vendors! And record everything you eat in your food diary.

Here are some good, easy, packable lunches:
- Lobster or shrimp salad with no-oil vinaigrette (see recipe)
- Chicken salad made with no-oil vinaigrette (see recipe)
- Pita sandwiches filled with tuna salad, no-oil vinaigrette (see recipe)
- Chicken with tapenade (see tapenade recipe)
- Cold shrimp
- Fruit
- Oat-bran muffins (see recipe)
- Cereal (the same high-fiber kind you would choose for breakfast)

I believe that spicy flavors make a dish seem more filling and I advise you to carry Tabasco sauce with you every day to spice up your lunches. Tabasco does contain some salt; if this is a problem for you, carry another spicy sauce or dry cayenne pepper.

DINNER

This advice is psychological, not nutritional, and it is different from what you might expect. Eat a lot of dinner the first night or two. Let yourself get full. Eat a few baked potatoes with your main course, if you have to. Eat spicy popcorn or potato crisps. Drink seltzer or diet soda. Go to bed feeling stuffed. Feel that you have no room for any more food. This will help to get you over the hump of the first days and nights, especially if you are used to crawling out of bed at night and rummaging through the kitchen.

For the first week or two, it is a good idea not to go out for dinner either at restaurants or at friends' homes. Commit yourself to eating sensibly, based on the recipes in this book. As with breakfast and lunch, record everything you eat in your food diary. When you do eat out, consult chapter 9 for help in dealing with restaurant meals.

SNACKS

Daytime. Snacks, fallbacks—whatever you choose to call them, they get you past the bad times. No one expects you to turn into a food saint overnight. You will get hungry between meals and you will crave your trigger foods. That is when my low-cholesterol fallbacks will help you immensely. When those crazy cravings overtake you, eat as much as you like of my potato crisps or spicy popcorn—they will be your bridge foods, taking you from your craving to safety.

And you can always snack on delicious fruits and vegetables. After exercising, I enjoy eating carrot sticks, although I certainly never stayed up nights fantasizing about them. But no one ever confused carrots with a trigger food.

Don't discount the satisfaction of a cold, low-calorie drink or a mug of hot tea or coffee.

Remember, snacks go into your diary just as full meals do.

Nighttime. At least for the first two weeks, don't have any snacks after dinner. (After that time, late snacks will become a lot less important to you.) Nighttime snacks used to be really difficult for me, because I started feeling deprived about 10:30 at night—not hungry, just deprived. I would begin to stuff my face and continue until I ran out of food. Then I would burp and go to sleep. Now I don't even think about eating after dinner.

If you can, say no, even to the usual "healthy" snack after dinner, such as fruit or vegetables. Once you have had your three filling and delicious meals, you would be better off with no snacks at all. The fact is, you are full. You don't really want that carrot stick, you just want something in your mouth.

MAINTENANCE

Many diets tell you to eliminate specific foods and then, as you lose weight, they put you on a maintenance plan, adding foods back little by little. There is no maintenance on this program. At no point will you go back to the foods you had to give up to go on the program in the first place. That would just be putting the needle back in the junkie's arm. But I promise you that the foods you eat will not bore you. I vary the spices, the preparation, and the combination of ingredients to keep you interested.

PLATEAUS

"Plateau" is a dispiriting word for anyone trying to change eating habits. You have hit a plateau when your weight loss levels off and seems to stop dead. Suddenly, you no longer see results.

When you are firmly committed to this program, plateaus become irrelevant because they have nothing to do with the lifestyle change we are talking about. Equally important, you are "counting" cholesterol as well as pounds, and as long as your cholesterol level doesn't rise, you are doing well. If your cholesterol does not go down to the recommended level through the combined means of diet and exercise, you should discuss this with your doctor.

Over the long run you will continue to lose weight, but you probably will reach a point where you level off. If this happens you have two options. You can simply keep following the program as you have been doing. After a time you will lose again, because *plateaus are temporary*. Or, you can actively attack the plateau by exercising more and/or cutting down on your food consumption. Just don't overdo either the exercise or the cutting down.

If you can afford the time and the expense, you can attack your plateau by getting away to a spa for a few days (see chapter 7). The experience will refocus your efforts and give you a concentrated dose of good eating and good living. It will most likely knock you off that plateau.

When that is impractical, do something on your own to break up your eating patterns. Look in your food diary and note what you have been eating for the last month—you probably have been sticking with a few favorites. For the next week, try totally different foods, different recipes out of this book, different preparations. Your change can be as simple as eating your normal dinner foods for lunch, and vice versa.

I give you a good selection of recipes in chapter 10. If you are like me, you will probably find ten of them that you are most comfortable with and you will prepare them again and again. But you can enjoy any of them, in any combination with each other. Don't get caught in a rut, eating your baked potato and roast chicken every night! Just move on to some of the other recipes. They all have the same focus, they will all help you to lose weight, and the change will energize you.

You can also change your patterns by throwing yourself into your work or into a new interest. I find that a long weekend in the kitchen of any of my restaurants is good for a weight loss of five or six pounds. It's a combination of the change of environment, feeding everybody else instead of myself, and the Exhaustion Diet I mentioned in chapter 3.

You will survive your plateau as long as you do not begin to feel sorry for yourself and backtrack. Don't give yourself the option of saying, "The diet doesn't work anymore so I will eat a pint of ice cream," or "I'm not losing weight anyway, so why bother to exercise?" We are not talking about fad dieting. You are accomplishing an overall behavioral change.

SUIT YOURSELF MENUS

I promised that you wouldn't be required to follow specific menus and I meant it. The combinations of foods and dishes you put together are entirely up to you: you can mix and match the recipes in chapter 10 to suit your own wishes. And don't stop with the dishes themselves—I want you to mix and match the ingredients of individual recipes, too.

Think about how you want to feed yourself.

Be aware of what you are eating and why.

Use the Yes list and the recipes in chapter 10 to devise your own delicious menus.

David's Delicious Food Program

SOME EXAMPLES

Let me tell you how two friends of mine put together a few of their meals when they started this program.

Laurie is a department-store executive who tried to stay out of restaurants for her first week. She managed to take her own lunches to work and she handled dinner dates by inviting friends to her apartment for dinner whenever she could. This is what she ate for her first week on my program.

MONDAY

DAVID'S BREAKFAST

LUNCH
CHICKEN SALAD SANDWICH ON PITA BREAD (NO-OIL VINAIGRETTE)
FRESH PEAR
CLUB SODA

DINNER
SEARED SHRIMP WITH STEAMED BROCCOLI
KILLER POTATOES WITH HOT CHILIES
GREEN SALAD WITH NO-OIL VINAIGRETTE
DIET SODA

TUESDAY

DAVID'S BREAKFAST

LUNCH
WATERCRESS AND ENDIVE SALAD WITH WALNUTS AND PARMESAN CHEESE
SPICY POPCORN
STRAWBERRIES
ICED TEA

DINNER
PASTA WITH GRILLED SHRIMP, LEEKS, AND SHIITAKE MUSHROOMS
RIPE TOMATO WITH NO-OIL VINAIGRETTE
FRESH PINEAPPLE
CLUB SODA

WEDNESDAY

DAVID'S BREAKFAST

LUNCH
COLD CHICKEN BREAST WITH
    TAPENADE
CARROT AND CELERY STICKS
OAT-BRAN COOKIE
DIET SODA

DINNER
WHITE BEAN SOUP
CRUSTY BROWN RICE WITH
    VEGETABLES
COFFEE WITH SKIM MILK

THURSDAY

DAVID'S BREAKFAST

LUNCH
LOBSTER SALAD SANDWICH ON
    PITA BREAD (NO-OIL
    VINAIGRETTE)
FRESH APPLE
OAT-BRAN COOKIE
COFFEE WITH SKIM MILK

DINNER
HEARTY TURKEY AND POTATO
    SOUP
LENTILS WITH VEGETABLES
CLUB SODA

FRIDAY

DAVID'S BREAKFAST

LUNCH
CHUNKY TUNA SALAD
SEVEN-GRAIN BREAD
FRESH PEACH
TEA WITH LEMON

DINNER
WHOLE-WHEAT PASTA ELBOWS
    WITH SHRIMP, CRAB, BLACK
    BEANS, AND PEAS
MIXED SALAD WITH NO-OIL
    VINAIGRETTE
DIET SODA

David's Delicious Food Program

SATURDAY

DAVID'S BREAKFAST

LUNCH
CANTALOUPE
WHITE-CLAM PIZZA
DIET SODA

DINNER
ROAST CHICKEN CHEZ LOUIS
POTATO PIE CHEZ LOUIS
ROASTED VEGETABLES
WHITE WINE

SUNDAY

DAVID'S BREAKFAST

LUNCH
ROASTED CHICKEN SALAD
SEVEN-GRAIN BREAD
FRESH GRAPES
COFFEE WITH SKIM MILK

DINNER
MUSSELS, SHALLOTS, AND
    CORIANDER IN SPICY BROTH
WATERCRESS AND ENDIVE
    SALAD WITH WALNUTS AND
    PARMESAN CHEESE
WHITE WINE

Starting an exercise program helped Laurie's resolve; she managed to fit in an aerobic class twice a week on her way to work and to take long bike rides on the weekend. She began writing in a food diary, too.

Elizabeth is a busy accountant who never likes to prepare her own lunch. She managed lunches during her first week (and some time after that) by stopping at a nearby salad bar and putting together tempting, low-fat combinations. She found salad bars to be real time and labor savers, and she was careful to avoid mayonnaise and rich but innocent-looking salad dressings.

However, Elizabeth loves cooking dinner, which she considers her therapy after a hectic day. Her first week's dinner menus looked like this:

MONDAY
CRISPY SCALLOPS WITH MUSHROOMS ON SPICY RICE
CHINESE GARLIC BROCCOLI

TUESDAY
WHOLE-WHEAT PASTA WITH TOMATOES, CAPERS, AND ONIONS
MIXED SALAD WITH NO-OIL VINAIGRETTE

WEDNESDAY
WILD MUSHROOM SOUP
ROAST CHICKEN WITH POTATO SLICES, TOMATO SLICES, AND GARLIC

THURSDAY
GRILLED SWORDFISH ON MELTED LEEKS
ROASTED MUSHROOMS AND GARLIC CHEZ LOUIS

FRIDAY
TURKEY AND/OR CHICKEN BURGERS
KILLER POTATOES WITH HOT CHILIES

SATURDAY
SEARED TUNA WITH MUSTARD AND ONIONS
STEAMED CABBAGE WITH SPICY BLACK BEANS

SUNDAY
ROASTED LOBSTER WITH TARRAGON
GREEN SALAD WITH NO-OIL VINAIGRETTE

Her desserts were always fresh fruit, berries, or melon, and her drinks were usually diet soda or seltzer.

All the suggestions above are not "meal plans" like those you might find in diet books. They are simply examples of how you can put together some of your meals, if you choose. They are not complicated menus consisting of many courses. I think most people are content with a vegetable or salad and a main course, or what I call "a vegetable and a hunk."

David's Delicious Food Program

And you can be unorthodox in your combinations. Many days my lunch consists of popcorn, and lentils with vegetables.

THREE GOLDEN RULES

Three rules go along with all this food talk.

They are equally important and interdependent.

You must follow them in order to ensure your success.

1. *Stay away from your trigger foods.* Every CE knows that certain foods will trigger an attack of out-of-control eating. Trigger foods will not satisfy your food craving; instead, they will open the floodgates to non-stop bingeing. Chapter 4 deals with trigger foods in detail.

2. *Keep a complete diary of everything you eat.* Recording everything you eat is an essential part of your psychological battle. (See chapter 8.) It is a strong, immediate way of monitoring your compulsion. It kills any desire to cheat, because you have to write down what you eat and then you have to face it in black and white.

Keeping a food diary requires that you take the energy you always devoted to overeating and channel it into writing. You will cut a track as you do this every day, growing stronger and stronger, and your control over your compulsion will increase.

3. *Exercise regularly.* I cannot overstress the need for a regular exercise program (see chapter 7). You will get optimal results only if you follow such a program. And the results and rewards will be measured by lowered cholesterol as well as weight loss. Maybe you think it is better to be on a diet without exercising than to be on no diet at all, but why not give yourself the maximum benefit available from a combination of the two?

Begin your exercise the very day you begin your diet and your journal. Don't wait. You may feel fat and ungainly, but this is all the more reason to get moving.

■ *Chapter Seven* ■

GET MOVING

Exercise is a combination of boredom and sweat. I have no secrets, no tricks to make it any more palatable than that. You can layer in all sorts of distractions; you can listen to music, watch television, or read magazines while you work out. But the sensible approach is just to admit to yourself that your exercise is not going to be particularly wonderful or intellectually stimulating or fun, but you still have to do it.

On the day that you begin this program I want you to begin exercising, because exercise is crucial to a successful diet plan. Even if you have not yet worked out a program for yourself, have not yet learned specific exercises or bought equipment, get moving in some way. Consider your exercise program to be inseparable from your diet; commit yourself to it and plan it out just as you do your food program. Prepare yourself to stick with it for the long run—one day at a time.

Because exercise is hard work and is often tedious, you shouldn't expect to love it. But you will grow to accept it because of its important benefits. If you are like me, you will pass through several levels before working out begins to feel good.

For the first block of time you will find it enormously hard to accept the fact that you must exercise regularly. Working out is painful if you are not in shape. You have no guarantees that it is going to help you, and you don't see any results yet.

But after a while you will transcend this level. You will find that you are becoming resigned to doing the work. You will see a little progress: you begin to lose some weight and your muscle tone improves slightly. You feel stiff after working out, and that is a good feeling.

You kind of bounce into the third stage, and then you are really moving. Exercise suddenly invigorates you and relaxes you all at once. The results are obvious to you and to others: your weight loss becomes visible and you begin to look trim and fit.

You have truly arrived when you feel that some form of exercise is an essential part of your day. On a day that you don't sweat, you miss it.

How long does each level last? I can't tell you. This is a totally personal journey. Your time frame is different from mine and from anyone else's. Get started and see for yourself.

I will not teach you how to do specific exercises in this chapter—there won't be any pictures of me in a sweatsuit. I will tell you about my exercise philosophy and my experiences and I will tell you where you can get exercise instruction.

WHY EXERCISE?

Of course you can follow the food program in this book without exercising, but the results won't be nearly as good. Here is why:

- Weight loss from dieting alone depletes muscle tissue. You don't want to lose lean muscle tissue, you want to lose fat. When you combine exercise with your diet, you will lose body fat and preserve lean tissue.
- When you exercise you speed up your metabolic rate and keep it

higher for some time afterward. So you burn up calories both while you exercise and after you have stopped.

- Exercise alleviates stress, works off anger, and promotes a feeling of well-being.
- For me and for many other people, exercise is an excellent appetite suppressant. I don't work up an appetite when I work out vigorously—exactly the opposite happens.
- Most important for me, regular sustained exercise can raise HDL cholesterol levels and lower LDL cholesterol levels. Improving my cholesterol levels was my original goal when I formulated this program.

Don't tell yourself that you are too busy to exercise, or too tired, or too old. Renee, a widow in her fifties, recently transformed her guest room into a home gym. She works long hours and also travels across the country as an executive for a computer company, and although she wanted to follow this program, she had trouble scheduling time for exercise. Renee felt a little guilty and extravagant when she bought both an exercise bike and a weight machine but, she reasoned, these were gifts to herself and she deserved them. Now her home gym has become her refuge. She works out every evening when she is not traveling and she has advanced to the third stage of exercising, where the results really show.

Margaret, who works in advertising, never exercised before she began my program. Now she reports: "David has me exercising! I go to a workout class four times a week. This is great for me because once I am in the class, I can't stop. I found one between the office and home, so I can't make any excuses. I also ride my bike around town a lot instead of taking buses or cabs. It means dressing differently, but I don't mind looking like a crazed middle-aged jock because I know it is going to change my life for the better."

REINFORCEMENT

Because exercise works as one part of a larger program, the principle of reinforcement comes into play. Regular exercise reinforces healthful eating, and vice versa. The stronger I become in my exercise program, the deeper my commitment to all the other aspects of my program.

ONE DAY AT A TIME

You know that more exercise is better for you than less (within reasonable limits), but there is no absolute magic amount you must do in order to lose weight and look and feel better. Many programs recommend that you exercise three times a week; nevertheless, I try to work out five times a week. My advice to you is: exercise *at least* three times a week. On the days that you don't go through a regular workout, be sure that you are active. Walk to your next appointment instead of taking a bus or cab, run around with the kids instead of watching them run, carry those groceries home, take the stairs instead of the elevator.

Make a decision to move around every day. Ask yourself, "Do I really have to drive there, or can I walk?" Remember that walking briskly is one of the best exercises you can do. You don't have to break into a sweat every time you walk, but you should be able to hear your heart beat and feel your feet getting a little tired.

And try to schedule your actual workout for about the same time each day you do it. This makes it easier for you to stay honest. It leaves you less opportunity to wiggle out of your commitment.

Remember, you are changing your life, not simply going on a diet. When you do all these things, each day means a renewed commitment to your new life-style. You must take the same responsibility for exercising your body as you take for what you put into your mouth. You can control your own physical state.

You are in this program for twenty-four hours at a time. You plan your meals one day ahead, you write in your journal every day, and you give up trigger foods one day at a time. Plan, each day at a time, to keep your body moving. If you can't bear the thought of doing situps or crunches into eternity, just concentrate on doing them this morning.

RECHANNELING ENERGY

Exercising every day is yet another rechanneling of the compulsive energy that usually goes into eating. (See more about rechanneling in chapter 8.) In my case, rechanneling has been so successful that I have to make sure that an exercise compulsion doesn't overwhelm me the way my eating compulsion once did.

It helps to make an effort to understand your own compulsive nature. For me, there is no letting my guard down. I know myself well enough to realize that if I were to break my exercise routine, it could have the same implication as taking one piece of candy. It might very well signal my first step into a binge.

But suppose there is an unavoidable break in your routine? I had to stop exercising for two weeks when I had a painful back problem, brought about by days of airplane travel. I had to take that punishing trip—there was no way out of it. But I could not resume exercising until my back healed. I knew that I wanted to keep my commitment strong and I worked on it. I told myself that soon I would be able to move around again. I didn't stop writing in my diary. I didn't bury my pain in an eating binge. I did not use my respite from exercise as an excuse to give up the program.

WHAT KIND OF EXERCISE?

Exercise burns calories, and I have always exercised—even when I was at my heaviest I managed to play football and baseball. So how come I didn't lose weight? Maybe you do the same thing and ask yourself the same question.

The answer is really very simple: the kind and frequency of exercise determines the benefit for you. Chasing a ball for a couple of hours once a week is fun, but it isn't done regularly enough to help much with weight or cholesterol control. And not only do you need the right kind of regular exercise, you have to combine it with a change in your eating habits. I may have moved around a lot, but I usually had a candy bar in my hand, which canceled out most of my activity.

AEROBIC EXERCISE

Back to the famous tick scare. When I learned that my life was in danger because of my cholesterol level and my weight, and I began to educate myself about cholesterol and diet, I discovered aerobic exercise.

The concept of aerobic exercise was developed by Dr. Kenneth Cooper and by now has become well known. By Dr. Cooper's definition, aerobic exercises: "stimulate heart and lung activity for a time period sufficiently long to produce beneficial changes in the body. . . .

"The main objective of an aerobic exercise program is to increase the maximum amount of oxygen that the body can process within a given time." Kenneth H. Cooper, M.D., *The New Aerobics*, New York (M. Evans and Company, Inc.) 1970, pp. 15–16.

Aerobics involves vigorous and sustained movement for twenty to forty-five minutes, so that a large amount of oxygen is pumped into the cardiovascular system. Aerobic exercise gets your heart rate up to a target number, which means that your heart is working faster. (I don't do it by the numbers, however. I have learned that working up a good sweat means I am at my best aerobic rate, and I don't bother to check my pulse.) When you exercise aerobically, your heart, lungs, and circulatory system get an extremely beneficial workout.

Aerobic exercise benefits metabolism and increases the oxidation of body fat; in other words, it helps you to burn body fat more efficiently. And, most important to me, aerobic exercise raises beneficial HDL levels and lowers harmful LDL cholesterol levels.

The general rule is to exercise at least three times a week. Some recommended aerobic exercises are jogging, swimming, jumping rope, biking, cross-country skiing, rowing, vigorous walking, and hiking.

I learned on my spa vacations that hiking is one of the best exercises you can do. A really brisk hike quickly gets your heartbeat going at an aerobic rate. I was never a runner, and most of my friends who used to run are now gimping along on bad knees. But hiking is simply a step up from walking. If you're hiking, you go up mountains.

Your aerobic workout should always begin with a five-minute warmup and end with a five-minute cool-down. The warmup will protect you from muscle cramps and pulls and the cool-down will help prevent muscle stiffness.

To learn about aerobics or to get yourself started on a program, I recommend that you read any of Dr. Cooper's books: *Aerobics, The New Aerobics,* or *The Aerobics Program for Total Well-Being* are among them.

You can also join an aerobics class at almost any YM/YWCA or YM/YWHA, community center, health club, or gym. Many useful classes are given at convenient times. I asked a friend to scan the bulletin of his local Y for exercise classes, and these are the offerings he reported: Coed Fitness, Aerobic Fitness, Slimnastics, Evening Coed Fitness, Weight Training, and Stretch and Strength for Healthy Backs. And for special-interest groups, there was an exercise class for pregnant women as well as one for senior citizens.

CALISTHENICS

Now that I am at fighting weight, I expect a call any day to challenge Mike Tyson. That is one reason I combine calisthenics with aerobic exercise in my daily workout.

You remember calisthenics—those horrible situps and pushups and leg lefts your gym teacher forced you to do. Well, they haven't gotten any better.

I exercise with a trainer and I know that every morning, no matter what, this person is going to come to the house and torture me. While I am exercising I concentrate on getting my mind out of my body. (That way, if my body is being tortured, I don't have to think about it.)

You can learn about calisthenics in the same way you can learn about aerobics, and in the same places. YM/YWCAs and YM-YWHAs, community centers, health clubs, and gyms. And, of course, in your library and bookstore, where shelves full of excellent, illustrated exercise books are easily available.

MY EXERCISE PLAN

My personal program, developed by my trainer, combines aerobics and calisthenics. It is divided into three parts. One part of the exercise is aerobic, targeted at getting my heartbeat up. One part is basic calisthenics—situps, pushups, leg lifts, and all the other things everybody hates to do. And one part is working with moderate weights.

I start with the exercise bike for twenty-five to thirty minutes. (The bike time includes my warmup.) Then I do stretches for five to ten minutes, depending upon how sore I am from yesterday's exercise. I stretch hamstrings, calves, waist, and neck gently, never abruptly.

After stretches I do a half hour of combined weight work and calisthenics. I combine the calisthenics and weights in either of two ways: heavy calisthenics with a little weight work, or heavy (meaning repetitive) weight work with very little calisthenics.

I exercise each separate muscle group. For the stomach I do crunches, situps, and bicycles. For upper body I do pushups. If you doubt the wisdom of these exercises, look at Herschel Walker. He got the way he is by doing a lot of pushups and situps.

For legs, thighs, and chest, I work with the weight machine. I prefer using a machine to free weights because with free weights you can sometimes hurt yourself if you don't have somebody watching you. A machine offers you a controlled range of motion. I believe in going for a lot of repetitions quickly. I lift a weight three times in increments of ten, fifteen, or twenty repetitions each. For instance, if I am doing 130 pounds of chest press, I will lift 130 pounds fifteen times, times three, and I will do it within five minutes. I never let myself feel strained.

I end with cobras, stretching everything.

If I don't have the trainer for some reason, then I do my own thing: twenty minutes on the bike, one hundred pushups, one hundred situps, weight work, stomach work, and stretches.

I look forward to each workout, demanding as it is. When it is over, I feel more relaxed and healthy than I did before I started.

On my weekends in the country, I'm always involved in aerobic activity. I'm sweating all the time, chopping wood, cutting the grass, building this, and tearing down that. It feels great and it helps to curb my appetite.

YOUR EXERCISE PLAN

I think my plan is best for me, but that doesn't necessarily make it good for you. If you want to research exercise plans, one way to do this (slightly sneaky, though) is to visit health clubs and be put through the paces of their exercise programs by one of their trainers. You don't have to buy, but be prepared to resist some hard sells.

If you want to hire a personal trainer, be aware that they can be expensive. You could hire one just for a consultation and start-up, or maybe you could put together a group of friends and share a trainer.

Once you have your program, or while you are in the process of creating one, follow the rules about beginning with a warmup, proceeding to a stretch, then using the separate muscle groups in their turn, and ending with a cool-down.

Use several kinds of exercise to condition every part of your body. But don't make the mistake of getting caught up in perfection. Don't try to give every muscle in your body the perfect amount of exercise. This can make you as crazy as calorie-counting makes you, and can turn you off the program completely. Gloss over it and get sweaty.

You can tell if a specific exercise is doing anything for you or if it is a waste of time. If you feel nothing is expanding, nothing is contracting, nothing is happening, or if you feel awkward, then go on to something else. If the exercise is right but you are not sweating, then you are not really doing it. You should hear your heart beat and feel your muscles burn a little bit.

EXERCISE AT HOME

Exercise classes often are convenient if you live in a big city—remember my friend Margaret who scheduled four classes a week between work and home?

But you don't have to be tied to a class schedule or to a bus schedule or to anyone else's schedule if you don't want to be. And you don't have to factor in travel time if hours are precious to you.

You can exercise indoors at home, as I do, using any of the excellent stationary bikes, rowing machines, or cross-country ski machines available. When you use them you cut down the inevitable boredom of exercising because you can read, watch television, or listen to music while you are exercising.

Some of these machines can be folded up and put out of the way when not in use; others just have to sit there on your floor. Don't worry about an exercise bike disturbing the design scheme of your bedroom—think of it as part of the design scheme.

An exercise bike is the single most important piece of equipment you can invest in. For exercise at home, in a small space, I rely on a stationary bike. Using a bike, you work up a sweat and get aerobic benefits quickly. Many people prefer a rowing machine or a cross-country ski machine; all are very effective.

It is worth the extra money to buy a high-quality machine, which may cost between $400 and $800. (If that sounds like a lot of money, ask yourself how much you have spent on candy and ice cream in the last year.) Good equipment is sturdy and easy to use, and not likely to cost you money in repairs over the long run.

There are many exercise videos available, aerobic and otherwise, that you can use at home. You can borrow or rent exercise tapes until you find one you can stick with and want to buy. On a recent quick trip through a video-rental shop, I spotted tapes on several levels by Jane Fonda, as well as the following:

- *Vital, Vigorous & Visual* with Joanie Greggains
- *Raquel: Total Beauty and Fitness* with Raquel Welch
- Callan Pinckney's *Callanetics*
- Kathy Smith's *Fat-Burning Workout*
- *Jazzercise* with Judi Sheppard Misset
- *Do It Debbie's Way* with Debbie Reynolds

For an even wider selection than your video store offers, you can order a free catalog listing almost two hundred exercise videos from Collage Video. Write to this address: Video Exercise Catalog, Department G, 5390 Main Street NE, Minneapolis, Minnesota 55421.

For exercising at home, get yourself a good mat and a slant board. If you want to work with free weights (I don't use them) you can buy one- and two-pound hand weights or dumbbells of three, five, ten, or fifteen pounds, and even heavier. If you are serious about weights and want to spend a good bit of money, I also recommend a professional weight machine.

EXERCISE ON THE ROAD

Many people who exercise at home or near home let it all go when they travel. Traveling doesn't mean suspending your exercise program; on the contrary, it means giving it a little novelty.

Even if I am only going away overnight, I pack gym shorts, sweat socks, a sweatshirt, and sneakers. I try to make sure the hotel has a health club or swimming pool, but if it doesn't I can still manage. I do fifteen minutes of situps and stretches in my room in the morning even before I have breakfast—the earlier I do it, the better I feel. I try to do something fairly strenuous every day: I will walk to a meeting instead of taking a cab. I've done pushups in airports.

I meet a surprising number of people who do the same thing. Jim and Fran, a married couple in their thirties, traveled to the Midwest for a family wedding and checked into a hotel the night before the festivities. The morning of the wedding they donned running shorts and T shirts, folded their formal clothes into their backpacks, and ran across town to the church. Once there they each ducked into a washroom, freshened up, and dressed for the party.

An avid exerciser I know gave his wife and friends a scare on a trip through Egypt. His party was waiting for a small boat to take them across a lake to a historical site when they noticed that he was missing. They were frightened, fearing the worst had befallen him in this strange country. But he appeared, huffing and puffing and happy, shortly after the boat arrived. Rather than stand around waiting and absorbing Middle Eastern atmosphere, he had grabbed the opportunity for a short run into the countryside. And once he stepped onto the boat, he found an empty spot on the deck and did some situps. The other passengers, mostly Egyptian farmers, were intrigued by this strange American custom.

WHY I LOVE FAT FARMS

To a compulsive eater it seems that no matter where you live in this country, someone or something is trying to feed you. Temptation is all around—on billboards, on television, in newspapers and magazines. Going to a spa ("fat farm" is the old-fashioned name) transports you into a clean environment for a time. You can forget the food-crazy world and concentrate on dealing with your habit.

Many spas are expensive, but if you are going to take one vacation a year, isn't it a good idea to spend the money on promoting a healthy life-style? Isn't exercising and eating healthful food preferable to lying in the sun and overeating (the usual vacation activities)? I believe that you can find a relatively reasonably priced spa if you shop around. Talk to a travel agent who specializes in spa vacations and read some of the spa guidebooks in your library or bookstore. Your research will be rewarded.

When I am at one of my favorite spas I stay in constant motion, sweating all day and feeling healthy. On a typical day I wake up early, at about 5:30. I go on an early morning hike, usually up a mountain, for about an hour, and then I come back for breakfast. I have some whole-grain cereal, fruit, and coffee, and then I am off again.

At 8:00 A.M. a series of classes begins, each class lasting forty-five minutes. I usually attend several exercise classes involving floor exercises or weights and a sports class, such as volleyball, before I break for lunch.

Lunch is lean, consisting of salad, fruit, cold soup, iced tea, and whole-grain bread. After lunch, I take a half-hour or forty-five-minute break before I resume my activities.

My afternoon exercises are more strenuous than those I do in the morning. They consist of heavy weight training and aerobic circuit training. Then I can slow down with yoga or a swim, followed by some time in the steam room or whirlpool. By the time I have done all this, it is 6:00 P.M. and I drag myself back to the room and get ready for dinner at 7:00.

Dinner is usually salad, a small portion of chicken or fish (sometimes a little beef is served, but I don't eat it), vegetables, and baked potato or rice. There is crunchy whole-grain bread, and some sort of fruit-based dessert. After an active spa day I feel tired and content, and I go to sleep early.

The spa experience is more than the sum of its parts—exercise, healthful food, and "getting away from it all." It can be a safety net when I fear I am going to get into trouble. If I feel seriously tempted to go back to the frozen Snickers bars, I try to get away to a spa, even for a weekend. It is like getting on base in baseball—it is getting into a safe zone.

COMPULSIVE PEOPLE BEWARE

A final caveat. Earlier I mentioned the possibility of overdoing exercise and turning it into another addiction. We compulsive people should be on guard against a transfer of compulsion, a growing feeling that we *must* do more and more exercise, increasing the amount daily.

Get Moving

If you do twenty sit-ups today, don't feel you must do forty tomorrow. The new compulsion will become as dangerous as the old one was. I have met real gym rats who exercise six hours a day, every day of the week. Sooner or later (if they live) that will blow up in their faces and they will fall back to doing no exercise at all. Try to reach a level of moderation.

Exercise is a vital tool for you to use in changing your life-style and improving your health. Try not to press it into the service of your compulsions.

Exercise has proved its worth to me. It has helped me to keep my entire program together. It has made me fitter and stronger than I have been in years. And it has done its part in lowering my frightening cholesterol levels. I intend to keep moving.

Chapter Eight

THE NEW YOU: GUIDELINES AND STRATEGIES

This chapter is about energy: the enormous energy you have always devoted to overeating and the energy you spend thinking about food, dreaming about food, and controlling food.

Rechannel this energy and it will empower your life change.

I devoted an incredible amount of energy to my food habit. First there was the duplicity involved in my eating on the sly. For years, my wife, Susan, thought I had a metabolic disorder. She and I would sit down to a meal and eat the same amount of food, and yet I was a big, fat person and she was slim. Later she learned that I knew what the pizza was like at every pizza shop in our extended neighborhood.

I was also very skilled at eating off my wife's plate in restaurants while she was engaged in conversation and looking the other way. And when we went to Chinatown and were served family style, I managed to be quicker and stronger than the rest of the family.

Does any of this sound like you?

The New You: Guidelines and Strategies

My character hasn't changed. I am still an energetic compulsive person. But I have learned to apply my energy in ways that help me, rather than using it to destroy myself.

You may not be compulsive to the degree that I am, but you can still hate yourself and live the cycle of gain, lose, gain, gain, gain.

RECHANNEL

Changing your life requires a lot of energy, and fortunately, you have it. You proved your strength when you carved out a food style that continually challenged your own best interests. Now take all that power and rechannel it in a positive direction.

Don't feel helpless—you're not!

When I worked out my program, I found that I had to make four general, overriding changes in the way I lived and thought. Each involved a positive rechanneling of the energy I had used before to feed my compulsion. Follow my guidelines in making these changes for yourself:

1 Exercise regularly.
2 Keep a food journal.
3 Take one day at a time.
4 Feed others instead of yourself.

KEEP A FOOD JOURNAL

Keeping a food journal is not a new idea, but I have found that my way works, and I will show you how. I had often used some kind of a diary as an adjunct to my diets, and I finally perfected the technique of recording what I eat and using the record to help myself. I've used big books, I've used little books, I've even used loose pieces of paper. I finally settled on a skinny little book, 2½ inches by 7 inches, called the Per Annum, Inc. Manhattan Diary, available in many stationery stores. (I'm sure there must be an equivalent Chicago Diary or Los Angeles Diary or Dallas Diary.) You may want to buy one of these or you may decide to treat yourself to an elegant "designer" diary that fits in your pocket or purse.

I use the left-hand pages for my business appointments and the right side for food. I write very small and I use abbreviations, but there are only so many words I can fit into the narrow space. The size of the diary limits my eating because I have to stop when I run out of room on the page. This may sound like a gimmick, but I assure you, it is true!

When you start your diet and your exercise you must start your diary—immediately. Don't worry about recording the quantities unless you want to say that you had just a taste of something or that you really overate. Otherwise, assume your entries reflect your normal portion of food.

Begin in the morning by recording your breakfast, and then, later, record your lunch. See if you have a craving for a snack in between; if you do, write that down, too. Record what you ate if you gave in to the craving. Be sure that you write down all your temptations in addition to recording all the food you eat.

You will soon see that a pattern develops. You may learn that every afternoon at 4:30 you want something to eat. Does that mean you are hungry or just that you are in the habit of eating at 4:30? Will you really miss this afternoon snack if you give if up? By writing, you are learning about your habits and giving yourself a chance to work on changing them: that is, you are monitoring your eating habits.

Writing in your diary uses some of that huge store of compulsive energy you possess. You transfer the energy you have been using in eating to the writing and monitoring process. In my case, I've gone over the line and switched compulsions. If I can't write within fifteen minutes of eating, I become uneasy. In restaurants I often record what I have eaten before I pay the check. But no one seems to mind. Writing is a harmless compulsion compared to overeating.

The best overall rule I have found for resisting temptation and rechanneling eating energy is: *Don't eat that ice cream, write about it.*

The New You: Guidelines and Strategies

Mind Game: Work out a symbol or code mark for your food diary that represents "temptation." Every time you feel a compulsion to eat, put that mark in your diary. (Don't bother to record the food; concentrate on the compulsion.) For instance, you have just finished breakfast and you are walking to work. As you pass a grocery store, you see a display of doughnuts. Out comes the diary, while you sprint away from the doughnuts.

Count how many times a day you are about to go off the deep end. You may be surprised to learn that it does not happen as much as you think. And as you stay on the program, it will happen even less.

Of course, the major part of your diary will consist of what you eat, not what you resist. If you record everything, it will only take a few days for you to discern a pattern in your eating. And once you have done that, you will find it easy to begin to tailor your eating to fit your new rules. Soon you will take a lot of pleasure in reading over your day's or week's healthful menus.

MY JOURNAL

My diary entries are brief because so much is assumed and the assumptions never change. For instance, whenever I write "fruit" or a particular fruit like strawberries or pineapple, I mean fresh. Whenever I write "muffin" I mean oat-bran muffin; "cookie" means oat-bran cookie. Any time a meat or fish is mentioned it is assumed to be prepared without fat, unless I also write "olive oil." Mussels are assumed to be steamed. "Coffee" means coffee with skim milk, unless it is "bl," or black. "Wh" is white, as in white wine. "Cereal" or cereal by name means with skim milk. The only cheese I eat is parmesan, and I measure that: "1 oz. ch." means a one-ounce chunk, eaten solid or grated. "Little taste of everything" is an entry I use when I dine with my restaurant-critic friends. It means that I didn't order anything for myself and that I tasted no more than two bites of each dish on the table—excluding triggers, of course.

YOUR ROAD TO RECOVERY

I use my own shortened words and simple abbreviations.

B = breakfast
L = lunch
D = dinner
chix = chicken
ob = oat bran
½ = ½ order
cant. = cantaloupe; ¼ cant. = ¼ of the melon, not ¼ order
/ = with or on (as: turkey/rye)
n.d. = no dressing (as in salad/n.d.)
sm. = small
sm. chunk = small chunk
veges = vegetables

Now that you know the code, you can read a few of my entries. They are for breakfast, lunch, and dinner—no snacks are included.

Monday
B. Strawberries, muffins, coffee
L. Mussels, ½ chix, salad/n.d.
D. Lentils/veges, salmon, red wine, ¼ cant.

Tuesday
B. Total/blueberries, coffee
L. Peach, 1 oz. ch., ½ cant., grapes, muffins
D. Turkey/rye, salad/n.d., pickles, apple, Diet Coke

Wednesday
B. Muffins, ¼ cant., coffee
L. Chix breast/tapenade/flat bread, peach
D. Salmon, wehani rice, broccoli, espresso

Thursday
B. Grapes, ob cereal, coffee
L. Lentil soup, cookie
D. Restaurant: little taste of everything

Friday
B. OB cereal/pineapple, coffee
L. Plate of fruit, muffin
D. Chinese food: shrimp/bl. bean sauce, steamed chix/veges, white wine

TAKE ONE DAY AT A TIME

When my eating was out of control I thought about feeding myself in terms of twenty-four-hour periods. I went to the supermarket and bought enough food for one day at a time. The expression "stocking up" was not in my vocabulary, nor was the word "leftovers." All you CEs know why I did this: if I had food in my possession, I had to eat it—all of it.

When I became determined to fight this behavior, I didn't discard my twenty-four-hour time frame, I rechanneled it. This is how I have changed.

Now, each day I consider where I will be for each of my meals and what I probably will be eating. I think about what kind of healthful lunch I can prepare or buy. I think about where I will be eating dinner, because that influences what I eat for lunch. If I expect to go out, or to eat a lot later, it isn't hard to eat less at midday.

When I face a trigger food, I find it easier to say no one day at a time than to contemplate saying no for the rest of my life.

I check off my day's exercise quota one day at a time.

Before I go to sleep at night, I plan the next day's breakfast.

You don't have to deal with your entire life all at once. If you think of this program in twenty-four-hour increments, *one day at a time,* each day becomes a separate goal. But each day will build on the day that has gone before, so you will find yourself "banking" these successful days and growing stronger.

I thought about food a lot when I was overeating and I think about food a lot now. I will probably always think about food. But the difference in my life is clear: now I plan each day to help myself.

Mind Game: Plan one entire day—how about tomorrow? Since this will be your first planned day, take a sheet of paper and write everything down (later you will do this all in your head). Use chapter 6 and the recipes in chapter 10 to plan your breakfast, lunch, and dinner. If any of those meals will be eaten away from home, follow the guidelines in chapter 9. If you know that lunch or dinner will be eaten out, make your other major meal porportionately lighter.

Write an outline of tomorrow's exercise. For instance:

- Walk to work—20 minutes
- Walk home—20 minutes
- Exercise video—40 minutes

List your triggers and promise yourself that you will not eat them for twenty-four hours. Don't think beyond that limited time frame.

Evaluate yourself at the end of the day. Were you able to follow this program for twenty-four hours? Remember, beginnings are the hardest, but they are possible.

FEED OTHERS INSTEAD OF YOURSELF

According to my mother, I am one of the lucky few who makes a living out of his obsession. (Who else does? Maybe a professional athlete.) There is no question that I always have been obsessive about food, devoting myself to finding or producing the best of everything. And I started out wanting all those cookies and cakes and ice creams for myself—that's why they had to be the best.

Now I am content with seeing other people enjoy fine food.

It helps to be in the food business if you are going to feed others instead of yourself, but it isn't essential. Most people aren't going to open a bakery or a restaurant because they want to beat their eating compulsion. You will find that in everyday life it is remarkably easy to feed someone else when you feel the need to overeat. And by taking care of other people, you will take care of yourself.

This isn't a new idea, by the way—many others have thought of it too. Karen has been a diabetic since childhood and can't

The New You: Guidelines and Strategies

remember when she last tasted chocolate, cake, or any other sweets. But she bakes fantastic cakes and cookies for her family and friends, and she positively beams when she serves all these delicious treats. She has a reputation as a talented and generous hostess, although she has never tasted anything she baked!

I remain obsessed with the best of everything, but I have rechanneled my compulsive energy, and it has made me a very fine host. Managing the food uses up as much of my energy as eating it once did.

Let me tell you how I spent a recent Thanksgiving. I had been invited to dinner that afternoon, so I got up early Thanksgiving morning and baked a delicious pie. I walked all the way to the dinner, about thirty blocks, lugging the pie (a little extra exercise never hurts), and presented it to my hostess at the door.

When I followed her into the living room, I immediately saw a huge bowl of caviar. I glared at it and thought, "You're not going to get me!"

Then I stationed myself by the bowl and made caviar canapes for the other guests. Whenever someone wanted caviar, I passed it out. I put my energy into feeding my companions. That accomplished, I promptly forget about the caviar.

I did the same with the pie. I cut careful slices, arranged them perfectly on dessert plates, and passed them out with great ceremony. My friends, being fairly normal eaters, could handle reasonable portions. I couldn't and I knew it.

I love to pick up food and poke at it, cut it up, arrange it. I feel that its okay to "fondle" food. CEs want to control that mound of whatever is in front of them. Eating it all used to be my way of controlling it, but now I love to make dessert, and sniff it, and serve it—to other people.

When I was younger, I wasn't so subtle. I remember sitting on my brother and forcing him to eat ice cream and cake. I see now that I was trying to transfer my compulsive behavior to someone else in an attempt to make it go away. Fortunately for everyone, since then I have refined my technique.

Mind Game: The next time you are invited out to dinner, offer to bring the hors d'oeuvres or dessert—in fact, insist upon bringing something. Once you get to the party, take charge of that food. Concentrate on using your energy to feed others instead of yourself. Enjoy managing the food and you won't have to eat it.

STRATEGIES

You know the overall rule, rechannel your energy, and the general guidelines: exercise regularly, keep a food journal, take one day at a time, and feed others instead of yourself. Now let's go to specific strategies. You need advice you can count on. You need everyday steps to take in changing your life. Unless you bury yourself in a cave you won't be able to run away from food. You will always be tempted. How do you deal with temptation?

In working out this program for myself, I developed practical strategies that continue to keep me on track. Like everything else in this book, they depend strongly upon common sense. They work for me and they will work for you, too. Here they are, simple and to the point:

1 Refuse harmful foods
2 Allow yourself food fallbacks
3 "Eat dinner" before you eat dinner
4 Build positive habits
5 Project yourself sixty seconds into the future
6 Talk to yourself
7 Talk to a food buddy
8 Go public

REFUSE HARMFUL FOODS

In the course of any given day, you will have to make many decisions about whether to eat particular foods. Decide beforehand that you are going to *refuse to eat harmful foods*.

If this is too overwhelming right now, decide that for the next day you will refuse five times in a row, or twenty-five times in a row—whatever you can handle. Just get it into your head that you will say one *no* at a time—you won't give in to one individual hunk of temptation. If you refuse a chocolate cream pie, that doesn't mean you won't accept an apple pie ten minutes later, but at least you haven't eaten that one thing. I guarantee that the more consecutive refusals you manage, the easier it will get. Start by saying no to five bad foods in a row:

- You are bored, you open the freezer, and you see an ice-cream bar. No!
- You are at a breakfast meeting and someone offers you a doughnut. No!
- A friend urges you to try a piece of homemade cake. No!
- The special pasta at lunch is fettucine Alfredo. No!
- It's your child's birthday and you are cutting the cake. No!

Be very aware of how you feel after you have accomplished each refusal. Do you feel stronger? Did the process become easier as you went on? Now try for another five.

There is a positive side to this negative exercise. It is all right to feel good about yourself—maybe even a little holier than thou—when you refuse harmful foods.

ALLOW YOURSELF FOOD FALLBACKS

You won't go overnight from being a devil to being a saint, so you have to *allow yourself food fallbacks and bridge foods*. If you are going to fall off the wagon, at least you will fall intelligently. My fallback foods don't make me feel I blew the whole thing and have to start all over again.

On this program you can nibble harmlessly on munchy-type foods:

- Potato Crisps (see recipe)
- Spicy Popcorn (see recipe)
- Sugar-free, low-fat, whole-wheat pretzels
- Bananas
- Grapes
- Baked potatoes

I don't mean to say that these foods are noncaloric. What I believe is that they are filling, healthful, and nonaddictive. Unless they happen to be your triggers, they will not set off a cycle of crazed overeating.

When I first began my program, I had to fight the feeling that I was "hungry" most of my waking hours. Spicy popcorn was my bridge food: it brought me from out-of-control eating to eating reasonably. I ate a lot of popcorn in the early weeks, but it gradually became less important to me as I simply stopped needing to eat so much.

At times you may eat too much food, even if the food itself is perfectly fine for you. But you know what too much is without measuring portions and counting calories. You know when you have pushed the limit just a bit too far, even if you have not actually binged. When that happens, fallback foods will help you to adjust your eating habits back to normal.

On a recent country weekend I ate too much barbecued chicken. I didn't eat any trigger foods and I didn't binge, but I had that uncomfortable feeling that I had gone too far. So for lunch Monday, back in the city, I had two good-sized baked potatoes. They put me back in control. They were satisfying, too, and I didn't feel that I was punishing myself for the barbecued chicken.

If you weaken, your fallback foods will save you.

"EAT DINNER" BEFORE YOU EAT DINNER

The same goes for lunch. If you expect to be in an especially tempting social situation, *eat something healthful and filling before you go out*. There is more to this than just getting yourself full. You will take control of a potentially dangerous event by taking control of yourself beforehand. You will prove that you are in charge of your eating.

You don't have to eat a lot at home to acocmplish this. I was preparing to go out for an elaborate restaurant meal with friends, and I wondered if I could resist overeating. I "ate dinner before I ate dinner," and at the restaurant I ordered nothing for myself and

The New You: Guidelines and Strategies

ate only a few tastes of dishes that were passed around the table. My diary entry for that evening says it all: "Snack: Baked potato/chix slice. Dinner: four tastes, white wine, did fine."

BUILD POSITIVE HABITS

When you repeat a positive action (such as saying no to harmful foods) again and again, you form new habits. It is almost like learning to walk and talk all over again. Practice that new behavior until it is natural to you. *Don't give up until it becomes a habit*.

Mike was accustomed to walking to the bus stop every morning, and then riding to work. Every single day for years he had stepped into a candy store for the morning newspaper—and a candy bar. It had become so habitual that most days he didn't even remember buying the candy, much less eating it.

Mike gave himself an assignment: buy a newspaper and don't buy anything to eat. This was easy to monitor—he knew he had an opportunity to repeat and reinforce his behavior five mornings a week. Every time he avoided the candy counter he felt he was changing a bad habit and practicing a new, good habit. It was gratifying to see a change in himself and to feel responsible for it.

Do you walk to work and pick up food along the way? Is the food you pick up likely to be a huge, sweet muffin or a bagel slathered with cream cheese? Compulsive eaters always seem to reach for something on the way to work (or on the way to pick up the kids, or while shopping or window shopping). This is a good habit to change. Even if you have to clock yourself block by block, walk to your destination without stopping for food.

PROJECT YOURSELF SIXTY SECONDS INTO THE FUTURE

I have told you that I think twenty-four hours ahead of myself. Sometimes it helps to *think sixty seconds ahead*. Suppose I am sitting in a restaurant waiting for the waiter to appear, and the fragrance of the fresh bread and butter overwhelms me. I want to eat the bread and butter—all of it. So I let myself imagine that I have already eaten it and I verbalize my feelings: "Okay, I've eaten this bread and butter. Did I need to eat it? Do I really feel better? No—I am mad as hell at myself! And it wasn't all that great. Was it worth the step backwards? *No!*"

TALK TO YOURSELF

Don't take your progress for granted. You have a decision to make every time you are about to eat a bite of food—any food. Even if it makes you feel ridiculous, *talk to yourself about each food decision*.

"I don't want to eat that junk!"

"I should eat breakfast. So I don't feel like it. I'm going to eat it anyway."

"Dope! Who needs that doughnut?"

The week of my fortieth birthday I spent a lot of time talking to myself. I went to a week's worth of birthday dinners and I had a wonderful time at each of them. In the old days I probably would have gained ten pounds celebrating, but this year I didn't gain one ounce. I wished myself a happy birthday each time I resisted a particular temptation, and I verbally patted myself on the back. And I ate very well at these dinners. I will tell you more about them in chapter 9.

TALK TO A FOOD BUDDY

Sometimes it helps to telephone or to sit down with a friend who is going through the same process you are. *Find a food buddy to talk to about your problem and its solution*.

Don't turn your wife or husband into your food buddy. Keep the buddy relationship strictly about food and make it the forum for all your food doubts and difficulties. Why impose those particular problems upon your spouse? Besides, if your spouse is not a CE, he or she won't understand most of what you are talking about anyway.

Early in my career as a chef I worked with a young woman who was fighting her food compulsion. She and I helped each other through many food crises. We each found the other to be a sympathetic friend, and we still speak to each other about compulsive

The New You: Guidelines and Strategies

overeating. Now both of us have very much more positive things to say.

What specifically can a food buddy do? My buddy says: "It really doesn't help to talk when you're in the middle of an attack. You feel such despair and misery that you just don't know how you will ever get hold of yourself. You feel totally alone. You need a confessor after the fact who can help you to feel less horrible about yourself. Just knowing that someone could empathize and understand made me feel better."

The buddy relationship was a little different for me. I did call when I was tempted to overeat. Sympathy and understanding helped me over the rough spots.

Building on a foundation of friendship, you and your food buddy can help each other to regain self-respect and begin to take control of life. There are some ground rules:
- You are there to help each other.
- You are there to reinforce each other in your behavior change.
- You are not there to link arms and run off to the ice cream store together—that's not what a food buddy is for.

GO PUBLIC

You can reinforce your decision to change your life if you tell the world about it. *Let everyone know that you are on this program—and then don't let them down.* Sometimes it is easier to live up to others' expectations of yourself than it is to meet your own. And support is vital. Your family, spouse, girlfriend, boyfriend, or roommate can be of enormous help. So bring your decision out into the open and get others caught up in it.

In the fall of 1988, a number of newspaper articles were written about people in the food business who were fighting overweight. A couple of stories mentioned me and my victory over my weight and cholesterol, and even included pictures. "I can't backslide now," I thought when I saw these stories. "It would be too embarrassing!"

If you don't have access to journalists and photographers, you can still draw attention to your victory. Talk about your life-style change when you go out with friends. Don't worry about boring them—people who don't have to lose one hundred pounds nevertheless are interested in the subject of weight loss. A lot of people talk to me about cholesterol and diet even when I don't bring it up. Everyone relates to good health and longevity. These issues aren't fads and they aren't about to go away.

NO EXCUSES ACCEPTED

Boy, have I heard some convincing excuses for compulsive eating. Some of the best of them came from me, including the "Top, Side, and Middle Theory of Eating a Chocolate Cake."

"Not enough time" is one of the most common excuses for eating compulsively and it is easily disposed of. I believe you when you say that you have a busy life, an aggravating life, with too much to do and not enough time to do it in. I know that changing the foods you eat and the way you prepare them will take some time initially. But either you make a decision to change your eating style or you will spend the rest of your life stopping the car in front of pizza parlors—which takes time, by the way.

Here are a few of the classic apologies for stuffing your face:

- I'll never get to eat this again. The world is going to end tomorrow and I will have missed this fried chicken.
- I'm here (on this island, on this cruise ship, at this Thanksgiving dinner). What can I do?
- How can I study (sleep, work, cook) on an empty stomach?
- I am in the food business, so I have to taste everything. This is a part of my education.
- That cake looks a lot like the ones I bake and sell. I'd better taste it to make sure the chef isn't ripping off my ideas.
- I may want to go into the food business. How will I ever get anywhere if I don't taste things?
- I'm uncomfortable. I didn't want to come to this party in the first place. No one here is interesting. I'm not interesting. Only the food is interesting.

The New You: Guidelines and Strategies

- I wonder what this tastes like.
- I bet this will taste awful.
- I wonder if I can eat just one.
- I have to take my medicine on a full stomach.
- I can always start my diet on Monday.

Here is my considered, in-depth answer to all of the above: *Just who do you think you are kidding?*

■

Now put all this together and go forth into the real world. You can face restaurants, dinner parties, buffets, ball games, and plane trips and still remain on this program. And you can have a lot of fun while you do it.

Chapter Nine

NOTHING BUT THE BEST: EATING AWAY FROM HOME

When I was a student I spent five consecutive summers in France, dining again and again at the Restaurant Troisgros in Roanne. I loved cooking and I desperately wanted a job in that restaurant's kitchen—I was like the computer whiz kids who understand programming but want to take apart the machine to see how it works. I finally got my chance after law school, when I was granted a job at Restaurant Troisgros and was then promoted to *cuisinier*. I learned nearly everything about how a fine kitchen functions.

I tell you all this because I want you to take the advice I give in this chapter. You can eat restaurant meals on this program! I know restaurant kitchens intimately and I know that they can accommodate your needs.

RESTAURANT DINING

Restaurants can sabotage you with temptations that begin with

Nothing But the Best: Eating Away from Home

the bread and butter and continue through the dessert. But you can outsmart temptation—I'm going to tell you how.

The key is: *put yourself in charge of what you eat.* Once you are in charge, you won't have to worry about restaurants undoing all your good work. Part of being in charge is realizing that you do not have to order an appetizer or soup, a main course, a salad, a dessert, and coffee. There is nothing wrong with having only a main dish, or only an appetizer, or perhaps an appetizer and a salad. Then you can go straight to your coffee or tea. Just because you are in a restaurant, don't feel that you have to order every course.

Another part of being in charge is the freedom not to eat all the food you are served. CEs often feel compelled to "clean their plates," so when you hear that shadowy voice from the past urging you to eat, destroy the food before it destroys you. Pour water on it, empty the salt-shaker all over it. Stay in charge of that food.

Throughout this book I urge you to throw away food rather than eat it. "But how can I waste food, how can I be so selfish?" you may ask. It is not easy to go against the values you were taught as a child, the values that shape your life as an adult. But as a compulsive eater you have been misusing those values. They are not an excuse to stuff yourself beyond the point of reason. When it comes down to a choice between harming yourself by overeating and throwing away good food—even though people all over the world are starving—you are in an emergency situation. First, save your life. Then you can proceed to live rationally.

Having given you these overall guidelines, I offer you four specific rules for restaurant dining. They are motivated by common sense and by your commitment to eating the right foods. And they work

1 "Eat dinner" before you eat dinner.
2 Talk to the waiter.
3 Know which foods you intend to eat.
4 Exert some control over food preparation.

BEFORE YOU EAT

Eat a little dinner or a little lunch before you go out to eat. When your eating was out of control, this was called "taking the edge off" and it involved some kind of massive, unhealthy snack. Now it is sensible and it will help you to stay in control.

You may want to have something filling, like a baked potato or popcorn, or something that is just satisfying enough to prevent panic, like fruit. Do you remember my diary entry in Chapter 8? "Snack: Baked potato/chix slice. Dinner: four tastes, white wine, did fine."

When you eat a little dinner before eating dinner, you will go out to eat without feeling frantic about what awaits you in the restaurant and about how long you will have to wait for it. And you won't feel the need to eat everything in sight as soon as you sit down.

Once you arrive and are seated, it is perfectly all right to eat some bread—just do it David's way. This is exactly opposite to Mom's way: I'm telling you to "play" with your food. Pull the crust off the bread and leave the middle somewhere. Eat only the crust and eat it slowly. It requires more time and effort than the rest of the bread, and you will be working for your food. The crustier the bread, the better—texture is important. Suppose your meal is late and you sit there tempted by that chewy, soft middle. Pour salt on it, or pepper, or water. Destroy it.

Bread is fine as long as you don't eat it with butter—if the others at your table don't mind, you can ask the waiter to remove the butter. Remember that you are not going to eat bad foods. Here, this means: "I'm not going to eat the butter, but I'm going to eat some bread."

TALK TO THE WAITER

A good restaurant will give you what you want if you talk to the waiter or the captain or even to the chef. "The customer is paying your salary" is a dictum of the restaurant business. The customer is usually right. I know, I've been on both sides.

Often your best bets are "sympathetic" restaurants that serve lighter food—they may call it club cuisine or light cuisine or spa cuisine. When you eat in one of these places, you are spared the trouble of conferring with the waiter and planning what will go into the dishes you order. While talking to the waiter is a perfectly fine way to do things, you may prefer to say simply, "I'll take the club cuisine, please."

This food will be vastly superior to the diet food offered even a short time ago in many places. If a restaurant doesn't have a lot of experience in this kind of food, it sometimes may err on the side of caution and serve food that is too bland. Travel with your own small bottle of Tabasco sauce and you can correct that error. Or, since most restaurants have Tabasco, you can opt to ask for it instead of carrying it.

KNOW WHICH FOODS ARE OKAY

When you read the menu, don't look for dishes, look for foods. Think: "What do I want to eat tonight?" See what the restaurant offers in terms of basics. Which vegetables are on the menu, and what goes into the salads? What types of pasta are offered? Would you like fish, or shellfish, or chicken? See what kinds are listed.

Decide what you want to eat and then think about preparation. You can then establish your ground rules with the waiter.
1 You want the chef to broil, bake, roast, or poach food.
2 The chef can use a little olive oil, but no butter or cream.
3 The chef cannot include any of your personal trigger foods.

This isn't as difficult as it may sound. The issue simply is to get the kind of food you can eat on this program.

EXERT SOME CONTROL

Let's talk about the menu course by course, bearing in mind that you are free to order only one dish, if you choose.

For the first course, you are probably a little tired of that dieter's standby, salad. Are their other possibilities? If the restaurant offers quail, ask if the kitchen can grill one with just a touch of olive oil and serve in on a bed of lentils or rice. Perhaps the chef will grill mushrooms or some other vegetables. A half-order of pasta, prepared with very little olive oil, is another good starter. A first course of fruit is always a good idea—borrow from the dessert menu, if you have to. If you do want a salad, request your vinaigrette on the side and sprinkle it on sparingly.

If you would like soup, ask for consommé or a light broth, perhaps with julienned vegetables. If salt is a trigger for you, make sure the soup is a low-salt preparation.

Now to your main course. The scallops look good, but they are sautéed, fried, or broiled with butter. Ask if the chef can broil them with just a bit of olive oil or if he can poach them and serve them a la nage, in a reduction of their poaching broth.

If you are considering fish, think broiled, poached, steamed, or grilled. If chicken or game birds tempt you, add roasting (with very little or no olive oil) to this list of methods.

Straightforward food like broiled fish or roast chicken is easy to order. The real challenges are the very interesting dishes on the menu. If you want them, you have to control what goes into them. When you see a delicious-looking pasta, say: "Could you make sure the chef uses only a little olive oil because I'm trying to watch my weight." Or ask: "Can you have the chef make it low-cal by cutting down on the oil?" If you order a lobster dish, you can ask the waiter not to bring the roe, which is high in cholesterol.

Lobster and crab are good dining choices because they take some effort to eat and they will keep you busy. The same is true of clams and mussels, pasta, and quail and other small birds. You have to work a little to get the food.

When you choose vegetables, ask that they be steamed, or grilled with just a light brushing of olive oil. Try a baked potato plain or with salsa. Perhaps the menu will offer wehani rice, or another interesting grain, prepared without butter.

If you need something to finish the meal, order fruit—nothing else. My very strong advice is: don't mess with dessert! Eat your dewy, sweet strawberries or raspberries and feel virtuous watching the other people eat pastry. Remember the rule about talking to yourself? Just say: "No, I'm not going to eat that food."

WHICH CUISINE?

Maybe you go out for an Afghan meal once a year, but generally you want to stick to the most familiar cuisines. This is a good idea, because you can patronize a few known restaurants that understand how you eat and you can pretty well manage what goes into the dishes.

FRENCH

What is French food all about? Usually two things: cream and butter.

If you order the usual meal in a French restaurant, you will have an appetizer, a main course, and a dessert. How can you have these done your way?

The appetizer is easiest, because you can always get a salad (vinaigrette on the side), poached or grilled vegetables, poached or grilled seafood, or smoked salmon. In terms of cholesterol, you will be fine. If you don't trust the restaurant to follow your directions ("Just brush it with a little olive oil, please"), stick to the salad.

The main course is difficult; it is usually very buttery and very saucy. But part of the fun of going out to eat is seeing what the restaurant can do with a little bit of oil, and some spices, herbs, and garlic. Of course you can order grilled or broiled fish, but you can also try quail, poussin, cornish hen, or chicken. If veal is not one of your triggers, order it—carefully. Have steamed vegetables and potatoes cooked with a little oil. But be sure to ask about the potatoes because most French restaurants do them in butter.

Forget about any French desserts. Have the most beautiful, freshest fruit the restaurant offers, with no cream, of course.

Remember to talk to your waiter and to request firmly: "No butter or cream in preparation or at any time." Get it straight right away.

ITALIAN

If you choose to order a full meal in an Italian restaurant, you will get a little first course, a little pasta, a little main course, a little salad. A lot happens without your having to eat a lot. The range of dishes here is more conducive to dieting than that of French cuisine.

The beauty of Italian cooking is that it doesn't mask the natural flavors of foods and herbs. Marcella Hazan, one of the leading authorities on Italian cuisine, said that the secret to great Italian cooking is not what you put in, but what you leave out. To understand what she meant, order the freshest fish you can get, brushed with olive oil and roasted with rosemary or tarragon.

I prefer a grilled or roasted fish to one that is steamed, because just a bit of olive oil gives the fish flavor and a crusty texture. It doesn't make me think "diet food."

Italian chefs do wondrous things with clams and mussels. One of my favorite dishes is a white-clam pasta, made simply with clams, garlic, parsley, a little olive oil, good clam stock, and herbs. (A purist wouldn't dream of adding cheese.)

Pasta is my all-time steady, reliable, favorite order, and I eat it five to seven times a week. It gives me something to play with, it tastes great, and it fills me up. There are infinite variations on pasta dishes, and the best of them can be sublime. You can ask for tomato sauce or any other sauce without butter or cream and with a minimum of olive oil. Another standby is the crisp vegetable- or seafood-topped little pizza without cheese, or with just a little grated parmesan, that has become so popular.

Every Italian restaurant cooks with olive oil rather than butter. Just request very little oil in preparation (it is relatively high in calories) and avoid fat-laden cheeses like mozzarella.

The dessert rule holds here, as well: avoid complicated desserts and stick to simple, delicious fresh fruit.

Nothing But the Best: Eating Away from Home

CHINESE

Chinese cuisine is tough. If you don't believe me, just go into a Chinese restaurant and request your favorite dish made without any MSG, sugar, or cornstarch. And ask them to use very little oil. What comes back will not be the dish you had expected.

Every wok cook throws his signature ingredients into the pan in varying proportions, so it may be a problem to get things done your way. A Chinese cook may misunderstand your reasons for asking him to alter his recipes, and he even may be insulted by your requests. He has been taught to make each dish in a certain way, and if he changed it he would feel he was going against his training. Many Chinese cooks and even some waiters are not fluent in English, and communication can be difficult.

This doesn't mean you should avoid Chinese dining; you just have to focus. The relatively safe stuff to order is steamed, or left whole and indentifiable, like a whole roast chicken or fish. But find out if the "roast" chicken or fish you ordered is really deep-fried, which is sometimes the case in Chinese restaurants. If it is, peel off the skin. You can order almost any steamed dish and use soy sauce, or the sauce that comes with the dish, on the side. If you want soup, check with the waiter to be sure that it does not contain eggs or meat.

It goes without saying that you should stay away from crispy fried beef, fried dumplings, and fried eggrolls and spring rolls. Avoid the cholesterol-loaded ribs and the lobster sauce (which contains eggs). And repeat: "I do not want oil. I do not want sugar." If it comes out wrong, send it back.

JAPANESE

If you like raw fish, Japanese food is perfect. I always felt that sushi is not too bad if you cook it. Japanese food is praised for being low in fats and cholesterol, so try vegetables, fish, or shellfish cooked at the table in bubbling broth. The hand rolls are good; they are fun to eat and low in calories. And eat salads.

MEXICAN

You fool yourself with Mexican food. You say "Look at all these beans. Great fiber!" But the beans are fried in lard. And a lot of the food is chopped up and unidentifiable. Then you start drinking Margaritas, so it all goes to hell anyway.

Some of the better places give you "hunk food," my term for food served in pieces big enough to recognize. You can try the corn or flour tortillas, but be sure that they aren't cooked with lard. And if they are cooked with another kind of oil, ask what kind and how much. Stay away from the nachos. Salsa, made of tomatoes, onions, and chilies, is a good bet, as are grilled, skinless chicken fajitas. You can eat some grilled, broiled, or braised chicken, fish, and shellfish, but preparation can still be risky, so be sure to ask what goes into these dishes.

INDIAN

Indian food is delicious, but it is often prepared with ghee, which is butter. Even the vegetarian dishes tend to be greasy. Tandoori cooking, a high-heat variety of this cuisine, relies on very lean, grilled meat, seasoned with Indian spices. Tandoori chicken is a good choice, because all the fat, as well as the skin, is cut off before cooking. But the chicken is sometimes rubbed with oil before grilling, so find out what kind of oil is used and ask that the amount be reduced.

THAI AND VIETNAMESE

On a recent trip to Bangkok, I discovered Thai cuisine, which, if properly prepared, is a lot less oily and more spicy than most Chinese food. It offers delicious and greaseless clear soups, such as lemongrass, as well as many steamed noodle dishes. Coconut milk appears in some recipes, but there is so much to choose from on a Thai menu that this ingredient is easy to avoid. You have a large choice of fish, shellfish, and chicken dishes. You can also eat steamed vegetables, spicy cold cabbage in vinaigrette, and spicy pickles. The portions are small and you are served a lot of rice with each dish.

Soon after I returned from Bangkok I had a meal in a New York Thai restaurant that began with a delicious shrimp lemongrass soup. Two very good dishes followed: dry grilled shrimp and chicken with grilled scallions, and barbecued chicken with rice. The chicken was prepared using a mixture of powdered spices rather than a barbecue sauce. These oil-free foods had the clear, spicy flavors that are so much a part of my program.

Vietnamese cuisine, like Thai, serves wonderful appetizers combining small portions of highly spiced chicken or shrimp satays and fresh lettuce, carrots, bean sprouts, onion, and spicy red pepper. It is similar to Chinese cuisine in the way dishes are composed—shrimp with onions, shrimp with peanuts, chicken with peanuts—but it is lighter and spicier than Chinese. You won't find much cornstarch in either Vietnamese or Thai cuisine.

I haven't come across too many good Vietnamese restaurants in the United States, although Vietnamese is my choice for the lightest, healthiest Asian cuisine. And my experience with most Thai restaurants in this country is that food preparation is not as skillful as it could be and oil is often overused. Be sure to request very little oil when you order. Of course, you should stay away from any deep-fried foods and avoid the pork and beef dishes.

I think we may see more restaurants offering these two cuisines soon. I hope we do, because both can be excellent for this program.

COFFEE SHOPS AND DINERS

It is easy to eat healthful, American-style food at the urban coffee shop and at its suburban equivalent, the diner. Both places have a generous selection of dishes from which to choose. There are lots of fresh salads, fresh fruit, melons, and grapefruit. (Unfortunately, they probably will be displayed next to the lemon meringue pies and the custard puddings.) An order of roast turkey or roast chicken is a good bet, and there is often a broiled fish dish on the menu.

Soups can be good, but ask if they are greasy, or just look at them to find out for yourself. If there is grease floating on top, you don't want the soup.

Avoid the hot dogs, hamburgers, French fries, eggs, and anything with cheese or with oily dressings.

DELICATESSENS

A deli is a great place to go just to give yourself a shot of instant gratification about how well you are doing on this program. You may see a lot of big eaters doing themselves in with eight-inch-thick pastrami sandwiches, but you can say: "That's not me anymore."

My deli standby is a lean turkey breast sandwich, with mustard, often on one piece of bread. I like to slice a pickle thin and make it the top layer of my sandwich, instead of that second slice of bread. Or I can use a large lettuce leaf. Salads are good, and I even eat the coleslaw after draining out all the dressing.

Most delis do a good job of degreasing chicken soup, and I enjoy a big bowl without matzoh balls or noodles. It smells and tastes delicious, and everyone knows chicken soup is good for you.

FAST FOOD

I won't tell you much about fast food—it is a minefield. All I can say is use your common sense and stick to the salad bar; skip the greasy dressings.

The best fast food I know is not from any hamburger or fried-chicken chain. It is simply a portion of grilled chicken, eaten with a piece of pita bread.

YOUR WORD LIST

Here is a mini-vocabulary to help you order the right way in restaurants:
- poached
- a la nage
- roasted
- grilled

- broiled
- steamed
- vinaigrette on the side
- brushed lightly with olive oil
- paillard

How can you apply this vocabulary? Try asking for poached chicken, scallops a la nage, roast cornish hen, grilled tuna, broiled squab, steamed shrimp, seafood salad with vinaigrette on the side, broiled lobster brushed lightly with olive oil, paillard of turkey.

When you order this way, you are controlling what you eat and you are asserting yourself, instead of giving in to the impulse to eat every delicious-sounding thing on the menu.

ASSERT YOURSELF

If you plan to go to a restaurant where you have never eaten before, it is very comforting to call beforehand, ask questions, and even order your meal over the phone. Most restaurants will try to be helpful. Your dining companions will respect you for having this foresight and they will probably wish they had done the same thing.

Even at a restaurant that knows you, that has heard your requirements before, say something to the waiter, just in case of the one-in-a-thousand chance that the chef will use butter or some other dangerous ingredient. Do whatever you can to stay away from the food that does you in.

More than once I have ordered lobster without butter or oil only to find it served glistening with some kind of fat. I simply gave it back to the waiter. If you make a request and the kitchen tries to circumvent it because they haven't paid attention or because the chef is a mini-dictator, it's okay to assert yourself and make a fuss. It's better to be angry than fat.

If the chef insists that a particular dish requires butter, say: "What else can I eat here? If I can't get anything to eat here I will be very upset." It helps to express your feelings. It's better than rationalizing, telling yourself, "Here I am with people I like, I don't want to embarrass them, it's a nice restaurant, maybe this one time...."

"What about the people who invited me out to dinner?" you may ask. "I can't get angry at their expense." Yes you can! If you are in a tough situation and you have the choice of being socially acceptable and blowing your diet, or being impolite and walking out of a restaurant—walk out! Do whatever is necessary to keep control over what you eat.

But it may be a good idea to prepare your guests or your hosts for the way you plan to deal with the waiter. If you warn them beforehand, they are less likely to become uncomfortable.

LEARN FROM THE PROFESSIONALS

Here is a bonus piece of advice: when you are in a restaurant, eat like a restaurant critic.

A restaurant critic is one of a very special breed. Meal after meal, day after day, evening after evening, he or she eats out. And then he or she tells you, via the radio or newspaper or magazine, just how good or bad the food was.

If Critic A loves lobster and baked potato better than any food on earth, she may order it in the restaurant she is reviewing. But that is not enough for you, the reader. Maybe you are allergic to lobster and baked potato. You want to hear about the veal chop, the swordfish, the pasta primavera, the potato pie, and the tiramisu. And you want to know if all these dishes are as good at lunch as they are at dinner and if they are any better on Saturday than they were on Thursday. Critic A has to tell you—that is how she makes her living. Given this responsibility, it's a wonder that Critic A, along with all her fellow critics, isn't so fat she must be carted around in a wheelbarrow from restaurant to restaurant. How does she stay thin and still do her job?

In France, restaurant critics are rumored to have access to a magical pill that speeds food through their bodies undigested. They can eat unlimited quantities of fois gras and Chateaubriand, it is whispered, and not gain an ounce. I have never seen such a pill, and I am dubious. Anyway, in America, we do things differently.

I have friends who are food writers, and I will let you in on their secret. A food writer doesn't visit a restaurant alone. He or she travels with a group of up to six diners for any meal. No one duplicates anyone else's order, so they manage to fill their table with a wide selection from the menu: several different appetizers, soups, salads, main courses, and desserts.

The plates of food are passed around the table and everyone gets to taste everything. Our critic carefully tastes and evaluates each dish, but eats no more than a bite or two, even though the other diners may consume the equivalent of a complete meal. The critic is able to sample a wonderful bouquet of tastes and textures, but never takes the opportunity to overeat.

This method of dining can be a lot of fun. The next time you visit a really special restaurant with a group of friends, try it. It works for the professionals and it will work for you.

WHEN SOMEONE ELSE ORDERS YOUR MEAL

I went to a glittering dinner party given at a French restaurant, where the complete meal had been planned in advance by the hosts. Each table had a menu listing six things: an appetizer, an entrée, two vegetables, and two desserts. The entrée was red meat and every single thing on that menu was prepared with cream or butter.

I had my first real panic attack in months. I called the captain over and said: "I can't eat any of this. I can't eat cream or butter or red meat. I need fish! Broil a piece of sole with a little olive oil and bring me a salad."

I was sitting next to the actress Jill Eikenberry, who said: "I haven't eaten meat in nine years. I'd like what he's getting." The women next to her chimed in, "I want that too." A chain reaction went off around the table and everyone ordered fish and salad.

The captain pleaded: "I can't change the whole menu," so the others agreed to stick with the original meal. Jill and I got our fish and salad, and if looks could kill, everyone at the table would have done us in. They all wanted what we were eating.

Even when a meal has been completely planned beforehand, you have to try to substitute the foods you need. Don't be afraid that you will embarrass yourself. A lot of other people are probably thinking what you are thinking. Almost everyone today is health conscious.

HAPPY BIRTHDAY TO ME

The week of my fortieth birthday in March 1989 could have meant a feeding frenzy, a perfect excuse to fall off my program. A magnificent dinner party was given in my honor and I was also taken out to many gala dinners and lunches at my favorite New York City restaurants. My family and friends outdid themselves in planning elegant, sumptuous meals to celebrate my birthday in grand style. In the old, overweight, out-of-control days, I easily might have made that my last birthday celebration by eating myself into the ground. But this year I ate according to my own guidelines. Sometimes I ate full meals and sometimes I handled temptation by having just a few tastes of everything that was offered to me, except my trigger foods.

The first party was at the home of my friends Lauren and John Howard, and was prepared by Karen Lee. It was a delicious low-fat, low-cholesterol dinner consisting of my favorite Chinese dishes. I tasted or ate portions of a fat-free mushroom spring roll, scallops, grilled salmon with steamed spinach, roast chicken with rice and vegetables, shallots and green beans. For dessert I ate an extravagantly (but healthfully) poached pear.

The other nights I was treated to feasts at superlative restaurants. Here are some diary entries for that festive week:

Le Bernardin (tastes): raw bass, oysters, shrimp/vinaigrette, grilled monkfish/mushrooms, poached pear, white wine, espresso.

Nothing But the Best: Eating Away from Home

Le Cirque (tastes): skate, sea bass/ratatouille, scrod/truffle/artichoke sauce, crayfish/black trumpet mushrooms, raw tuna/yogurt, 2 bites fruit dessert, red wine, espresso.
Tai Hong Lauw: shrimp, oysters, clams, sesame chicken, noodles, greens.
Chez Louis: white bean salad, roast chicken, pretzel, red, white wine.
Mickey Mantle's: 3 chix wings (no skin), bean and escarole soup, flat bread, Margarita.
Pierre—"An Evening at the Hotel Ritz" (tastes): snapper, sole/artichoke/potato crisps, salad/n.d., white wine.

That week I celebrated a lot more than turning forty. I celebrated my new outlook on life, my low cholesterol, my lowered weight, and the prospect of a great many more birthday parties.

THREE-STAR RESTAURANTS IN FRANCE

You can order your own way in the most elegant restaurants. I have accomplished it even in three-star restaurants in France, and if you are planning a trip to France, you can do the same.

The captains in the finest restaurants speak impeccable English, so you can explain that you have a problem, that you can't eat certain foods. Ask what the chef can prepare for you. If you write to the chefs before your trip and make clear what you want and how you want to eat it, they will bend over backward to accommodate you.

Of course, they can't make you a fois gras with no cholesterol. You can't have steak buried in butter. But this doesn't mean you can't get something excellent to eat. A great kitchen should be able to turn on a dime.

Sometimes, though, it may take a bit of doing. When Susan and I dined at Moulin de Mougins, owned by Roger Verge, I gave the captain my usual lecture about what I can and can't eat and I proceeded to order. The first course was a lobster salad—just sliced cold lobster. Then came a vegetable dish, exactly as I had specified.

The third dish was quail baked in a potato with a sauce. I have enough experience to know when a sauce has butter in it, and Susan and I agreed that there was butter in that sauce.

"You must have brought me the wrong thing," I told the captain. "This sauce has butter." "Oh, no," he said. The chef had assured him that it was just an emulsion of port and stock.

I answered: "I'm a chef and I know exactly what's in this dish. If it contains butter I am going to die. I'm going to drop dead right at the table. It will be pretty embarrassing to the restaurant. Go back to the kitchen, look the chef in the eye, and ask him if he put any butter in the sauce."

The captain came back and whispered: "He put in a little bit at the end."

The quail went back to the kitchen fast and I ordered an excellent grilled sea bass with tapenade and tomato sauce, as a replacement. My diary entry for that meal concluded with: "I beat it!"

YOU CAN'T WIN THEM ALL

I have to admit that some situations are gastronomically close to impossible.

I went to a place in Nashville, Tennessee, called Opryland, a huge complex containing a hotel, convention hall, and ten restaurants. It is like a city within a city. I thought that it would be easy to eat reasonably there, but everything I saw in every one of those restaurants was fried or slick with grease. The shrimp and chicken salads were drowning in mayonnaise. I ran from restaurant to restaurant looking for something that wouldn't throw me off my program. As I looked around, I felt as if I was in a nightmare where everybody was fat.

I couldn't get off the property—there are no sidewalks leading out. I managed to climb a fence and cross the highway to a fast food restaurant, but the food there was 100-percent fried. I found a Seven-11 store and looked for some popcorn, but the only popcorn they had was full of coconut oil. I staggered back to the hotel and called room service. I told them that I had a medical problem and I needed baked potatoes. In a hotel with two thousand rooms the kitchen didn't have any baked potatoes!

I finally negotiated some gumbo that the kitchen staff swore had no cream or butter in it. Then I ordered two shrimp cocktails and put the shrimp in the gumbo, for a makeshift meal.

I wish I had called ahead on that one.

DINNER PARTIES

In the middle of one of my early, doomed diets, I went to a party in California given by Stacy Winkler and her husband, actor Henry "The Fonz" Winkler. Stacy is a phenomenal cook and hostess. She had invited forty people to this dinner and it seemed to me that there was enough food for four hundred!

I saw bowls of caviar, several different kinds of sausages, Greenberg's cookies and brownies, and just about everything else I had ever wanted to eat. That party, in August, triggered an eating binge that lasted until the following December.

Last year, after several months on my program, I was invited to another event at the Winkler house, but it was a very different experience. When I accepted the invitation, I told the hostess about my diet. I ate dinner before I ate dinner. I looked all that food in the eye and refused anything that was bad for me. Nobody made a fuss.

It can be difficult for CEs and recovering CEs to manage dinner at a friend's home. I attended another dinner party when I had been on this program for only a few weeks. The hostess enthusiastically served everyone a beautiful, rich chocolate cake for dessert. She urged me to eat some, saying: "You have to try this—it's my favorite cake!" My answer was, "I'm trying to lose weight. I can't eat chocolate cake." She persisted: "Just take a bite."

Now "just a bite" of chocolate cake, which happens to be another trigger food, would have undone me, as any CE can tell you. Then this woman actually tried to stick a piece of cake in my mouth. I had the terrible feeling that there was no place to hide. I felt as if I was dodging that cake, open-field running, as in a football game.

I declined quite a few invitations after that experience.

Since that time, I have learned to handle myself better. Let me share the rules that have helped me.

1. Tell the host or hostess beforehand that you are seriously working on your eating habits. Tell him or her what you can and cannot eat. Offer to bring your own food.
2. Eat dinner before you eat dinner. (It works here, too.)
3. Stick to your guns and don't worry about hurt feelings. Your host's hips, thighs, or arteries are not at stake, but yours are!

THE HOST'S POINT OF VIEW

A *New York Times* article quotes Charlotte Ford, the etiquette authority, as being "incensed" when a guest called her before a party to ask what she would be serving. Ms. Ford instructs: "If you don't eat certain foods, eat at home. Don't call up the hostess and imply that she should cook something else."

My attitude is different. I say, by all means call your hostess. That is better than sitting at the dinner table in a cold sweat. If you like, you can offer to bring some of your own food. (Although I really think that someone who cared to invite you in the first place wouldn't mind serving you something you can eat. I know I would be happy to do it.)

I agree that you should eat at home, but eat there before dinner, not instead of dinner.

BUFFETS AND OTHER OBSTACLE COURSES

If I have one skill in life, it is stacking pounds of food architecturally on a little plate. As a practicing CE, I developed a method that allowed me to expand the capacity of those inadequate six-inch plates you find on buffet tables. My idea was to build a support system that would expand the lower perimeter of the plate beyond its boundaries.

Nothing But the Best: Eating Away from Home

I began with bones—rib bones or chicken bones or, alternatively, chicken on skewers. Starting from the center of the plate, I fanned them out so that they extended all around. Then I proceded to balance them by stacking a pile of fairly dense food on top of the bones. Shrimp was my favorite choice. Having built this support of bones and shrimp, I could then layer other foods on top. I piled on fried wontons or sausages as I began to build upward. There was room for almost every kind of food on the table!

Eating took some skill. I had to eat down from the top in layers, just as I had built up to the top. Tasting a little bit of this and that might send the whole structure tumbling. So I was careful to eat from the top down until I reached the shrimp. Once the shrimp were finished, of course, the bones started to fall off the plate. Then I had to eat the ribs or chicken very fast.

When I face a buffet table now, I forget about structural engineering. I recently went to a dinner at my daughter's school, where the serving table was spread with temptations donated by the parents. Fortunately, someone had prepared a tray of spicy barbecued chicken. I helped myself to this good food and made it through the evening.

I behaved in a similar way at the latest CityMeals-on-Wheels dinner. Every year, some of the country's most interesting chefs present a dazzling evening of wonderful food for the benefit of this New York charity. I had a fine time admiring and sniffing their offerings. My dinner consisted of three little dishes: a small piece of grilled squab breast, two skewers of grilled salmon, and a slice of smoked fish. You may not think that constitutes a banquet, but I loved every bite, and I didn't let the richer offerings throw me off course.

If you are planning to go to a buffet dinner, it may be hard to control what you will be served, so be sure, as always, to eat extra dinner before you go out, because you are facing a perilous situation. Then, search the buffet table carefully until you find the kind of food you can eat. There is bound to be at least one dish. Zero in on it and eat hearty.

SPORTS FOOD

How can you separate the ball game from peanuts and Cracker Jacks—let alone hot dogs, beer, ice cream, soda, pizza, and candy bars? Is anyone in the stands *not* eating? The wonderful smells and tastes are part of the excitement of a day or evening at the stadium.

For some people, nothing could be more fun. And if you are one of these sports fans, I won't spoil your outing. But I will tell you to *bring your own food*.

Enjoy spicy popcorn, potato crisps, and all the other delicious non-trigger snacks you eat at home. They are portable. Stay away from the high-calorie, high-cholesterol foods prepared at the stadium. Eating this food does not have to be part of the sports experience.

Sure, the smells around you will seem intoxicating. But the things you have brought from home are just as tempting. And when you think of the fats, salt, and preservatives in those oily franks and greasy chips, your light, spicy popcorn becomes even more appealing.

Don't limit yourself to snacks, either. Bring a tempting picnic from home that will make the people sitting near you envious. Buy some delicious Middle Eastern flatbread, or if you can't find that, buy some pita. Make a sandwich of sliced chicken sausage (this sausage is available in supermarkets and contains no fat or pork) and spread the sausage with my fragrant tapenade. Sliced chicken breast is good prepared the same way. How about a salad of spicy black-eyed peas, and luscious fresh peaches or berries? Go all out. Being on this program does not mean depriving yourself.

Be extra careful when you get up to stretch your legs and walk around the stands. Snack bars and ice-cream carts are everywhere, calling to you. Don't answer.

A friend of mine went to the racetrack with her husband on a beautiful Saturday in June when she had been on my program exactly one week. Between the front entrance and her seat she passed stands selling hot dogs, pizza, Haagen Dazs bars, Oriental food, soft drinks, beer, and candy. She survived this onslaught by bringing her own fruit and munching on it whenever temptation threatened.

They spent the day in the restaurant overlooking the track, with a congenial group of friends who loved good food and drink. But sitting at a dining table all day didn't overwhelm her. In fact, she joined right in. She decided that alcohol wasn't worth the calories, so her drinks were iced tea and diet soda. She chose her food carefully. ("Why didn't I order that?" her friends asked, when they compared their deep-fried crab cakes and their greasy beef with her delicate poached salmon.) As the hours passed and they lingered around the table, she popped an occasional grape.

She had a delightful day and she came out ahead.

Most stadiums, ball parks, and racetracks have elegant restaurants or clubs like the one my friend enjoyed, where the well-dressed fans can dine while they watch the event.

These restaurants may be larger than usual (they sometimes have to accommodate thousands of patrons) but they are still restaurants. You can still communicate with your waiter and control what you eat. You can find out what goes into each dish and what can be left out of it.

Ask how that breast of chicken is prepared! Too often it is fried and then drowned in sauce. And the salads may well be loaded with mayonnaise or oily dressings. But along with the ubiquitous smothered and deep-fried items, there is usually something good on the menu that is poached, or prepared with just a little oil. There probably is a large salad that you can order with dressing on the side. Don't look for dishes that are grilled to order. These clubs must prepare many of their foods beforehand because they serve on a very large scale.

AIRLINE FOOD

The first time I went to Canyon Ranch, the Arizona spa, I weighed over three hundred pounds and I was desperate to lose weight. So I decreed that my diet began the second I got on the plane in New York. (This is a variation of the 12:01 A.M. Monday diet beginning.)

I sat on the plane and watched the attendants serve all the food to all the other passengers and I did not eat one bite of anything. And it was a long flight. By the time I got off the plane I was a raving maniac. Fortunately, once I got to the spa I got some good healthful food.

I avoided the plane food because I was determined to diet, and I knew I couldn't if I ate what was served. But there are better ways than starvation to cope with airline food.

You can pick around what they give you and eat what seems to be grease-free, sugar-free, and somewhat real. This is not altogether a good idea, because whatever they give you will not be dietetic cuisine, and it will be hard to find any good parts.

When you make your reservations you can order a special meal of some sort—kosher, vegetarian, low-calorie, no cholesterol, or salt free. Probably you can work out something that isn't fattening and that will fill you up. That doesn't mean it will be good.

I strongly recommend that you bring your own food. Plan ahead so that you can really enjoy your meals. They should be simple, easy to carry, and delicious. On a recent flight to Australia, I brought along two roasted chickens and some excellent French bread. The trip was much longer than the one to Arizona, but I didn't feel sorry for myself. Most of the people eating the airline meals felt sorry for themselves, even if they weren't on diets.

Don't be self-conscious! People may stare at you and your food—so what? After all, they are strangers and you will never see them again. And it is more than likely that they are thinking: "Why didn't I do that?"

How about the trip home? Susan and I spent a week in Italy (very enjoyable, even without gelati) and when we were preparing to return to New York I realized that I hadn't thought about what I could eat on the plane. So I bought some fruit and a large loaf of chewy Tuscan bread. I cut the middle out of the bread and carried the shell with me. At mealtimes I nibbled on my own picnic.

THE PLEASURE OF EATING REDEFINED

All of this thought and preparation will add up to a new way of perceiving food. After you have been on this program for a while, you will see a real change in the way you relate to food and eating. This is the cumulative benefit that comes from rechanneling your energy and changing your food style.

You will find that simple foods with clear tastes (like the ones in chapter 10) become infinitely more pleasing to you than complicated rich foods. You will be put off, if not disgusted, by grease. You will find that smelling food is almost as good as eating it—especially if eating it hurtles you over the cliff.

PART THREE

COOKING WITH DAVID

■ *Chapter   Ten* ■

COOKING WITH DAVID

What is really good food, and can you eat that kind of food if you follow my program? What makes the food I prepare—and the food you will prepare—delicious and unusual? How does everything I have told you in this book so far translate into your daily life at the table?

The best food in the world is impeccably fresh and prepared perfectly simply! Roasted mushrooms and garlic as we do them at my restaurants, Chez Louis and Broadway Grill, grilled baby chicken stuffed with sage, grilled swordfish on melted leeks, wild mushroom soup, potato pie with clams and coriander—these are my idea of perfect dishes. And they are all on this program and in this book.

Restaurant Troisgros formed my approach to cooking years ago. Based upon my training there, as well as on my other experience, I wrote *Cooking the Nouvelle Cuisine in America* with Michèle Urvater (New York, Workman Publishing, 1979.) That book has served as a glorious inspiration to me. Its recipes are built on the principles I follow today, and I even include here its recipes for chicken stock and fish stock because I consider them to be state of the art. There is one major change in the body of my cuisine: in 1979 I cooked with butter, cream, and eggs, and today I do not. However, many dishes in the early book are perfectly acceptable, requiring only an intelligent substitution of olive oil for butter.

The recipes I give you are basically what I have been eating for the past two years on my low-fat, low-cholesterol program. They rely on the Yes list foods in chapter 6 and they do not require any ingredients from the No list. Yet they are not made-up, wouldn't-this-be-nice recipes. They are real dishes and they meet my high standards. When I am hungry, feeling sorry for myself, or I must have something satisfying to eat *now*, these are the things I prepare.

"Satisfying" is a key word. The dishes you eat on a weight-loss, cholesterol-lowering program do not have to be fussy, empty, and bland. My food is hearty and filling, as well as being interesting in taste and texture. The point of eating it is to feel satisfied!

YOU ARE THE CHEF

To be successful on this program you have to be in charge of what you eat. You are doing the shopping, smelling the strawberries, looking for the freshest and the most appealing foods. You are cooking the meals and giving yourself the things you really like. *You are involved in the whole process of feeding yourself from start to finish.*

The approach to cooking is more important than specific ingredients and detailed instructions. And my approach, as I have said, is that food should be impeccably fresh and prepared perfectly simply.

None of the recipes in this chapter will fail if your quantities are less than exact or if you change some of the ingredients. How spicy you want your food, or how crisp, or how well done depends on you.

I expect that when you go on this program, you will cook for yourself a lot of the time, so many of the recipes serve one person

Cooking with David

The recipe for Baked Potato with Salsa and Seared Shrimp gives you the quantities needed for one portion; so do the recipes for Seared Tuna with Mustard and Onions, for Spicy Swordfish, Grilled or Seared, and for Roasted Lobster with Tarragon, among others. But you can expand any of these recipes to serve eight, if you like.

As you begin to use these recipes you will see that they lend themselves to "mix and match" flexibility. For example, you can make turkey burgers or chicken burgers or turkey-chicken burgers. You can prepare the burgers with onions or peppers or mushrooms or even white truffles. For flavoring, you can add Dijon mustard or Colman's hot English mustard or green peppercorn mustard. You can use different vinegars, such as balsamic, Champagne, rice wine, red wine, or tarragon. It is easy to suit yourself.

In most recipes, I give the amounts of vinegar, oil, and mustard you are to use, although there is room for flexibility here, too. When I list "pepper" as an ingredient, I always mean freshly ground black pepper. How much salt and pepper you use is entirely up to you— every recipe calls for salt and pepper *to taste*.

SALT AND FAT

The issue of salt is a little complicated. Even in the recipes containing salty ingredients like anchovies, you have the option to season to taste. If you don't care for salty food (as I don't), if salt is one of your triggers, if you are at risk for high blood pressure, or if there is any other reason that you shouldn't use salt, simply *leave out the salt—it won't change the recipe*. If you like, you can make the dish spicy instead—include any salt-free spice you choose. I throw a little salt in the water when I cook pasta, but it isn't necessary to do this. I don't add salt to the water when I cook rice or potatoes.

Through years of cooking a lot of different foods and playing with recipes, I have not only come to use less and less salt, I have taught myself how easy it is to cook with only a small amount of fat, usually olive oil. Often my recipes call for steaming, grilling, or searing food, using little or no fat.

I find that a lot of restaurants overuse both salt and oil. I would much rather have the taste of a fresh-herb-infused chicken-based sauce than something salty or greasy. If I were asked to choose either a plate of Chinese Garlic Broccoli or a plate of French fries, and I knew there would be no negative consequences from eating either one, I would eat the broccoli. (I am not yet sure I could do that with fried chicken.)

HOW LONG DOES THIS RECIPE TAKE?

If you are like me, when you are hungry you tend to get frantic and you want to have your food ready to eat as soon as possible. You don't want to think: "Oh my God, it's going to take me three hours to make that!" because then you will throw away the recipe and call up the pizza shop. Many of these dishes will not take more than twenty minutes to prepare and some will take half that time.

Some special recipes will take longer. My recipe for French Bread Pizza Dough requires careful mixing and three risings. There are no shortcuts here. But once you prepare the dough, you can refrigerate it for up to ten days. With the dough on hand, it takes only minutes to put together a delicious pizza. And if you want your pizza immediately and you haven't made any dough, the pizza recipes are adaptable. You can spread your pizza toppings on a pita, on flatbread, or on French bread or bagel crusts.

The roast chicken dishes (Roast Chicken Chez Louis; Chicken Roasted on Potato Slices, Tomato Slices, and Mashed Garlic; and Roasted Chicken Stuffed with Grilled Shiitake Mushrooms, Deglazed with Balsamic Vinegar) will take over an hour from start to finish because of the roasting time involved. These are wonderful party dishes and no one can accuse them of resembling "diet food." Although they aren't recipes for immediate gratification, they are worth making because they are lean, aromatic, delicious, and satisfying.

Some recipes give you the options of grilling over a wood or charcoal fire or using another method, such as searing in a hot pan or broiling (for example, Turkey and/or Chicken Burgers; Spicy Swordfish, Grilled or Seared; Grilled or Seared Shrimp with Steamed Broccoli). While the cooking time is usually the same, grilling requires extra time for preparing the fire and waiting until it is ready to use. Grilling adds a special flavor and texture, but if you want to prepare these recipes extra fast, you can use an alternative method.

To keep preparation speedy, I suggest that you use a modified-prep approach to cooking: this means that you need certain staples on hand to use in the recipes.

You should have chicken stock and fish stock in your freezer or refrigerator. I give you my recipes for these stocks, which originally appeared in *Cooking the Nouvelle Cuisine in America*. If you don't have chicken stock, you can use a good canned chicken broth, or even a low-sodium variety. If you work with canned broth, chill it first so that the fat rises to the top and can be skimmed off. You can sometimes use commercial clam broth as a substitute for fish or lobster stock, but be aware that it may be saltier than homemade stock.

Where a recipe calls for beans, you can use canned beans, thoroughly rinsed. Goya is one good brand. Of course, you can prepare dried beans from scratch if you have the time to soak and cook them.

Have potatoes and onions available, as well as fresh seasonal vegetables. And if you have no fresh vegetables, frozen vegetables will do.

You can easily grow your own herbs at home, assuming that you have the light and a bit of a green thumb. Pick out your two or three favorite herbs and get a pot of each going in the kitchen, yard, or on the roof. My favorites are rosemary, sage, and chives. Some other good ones are tarragon, mint, and basil. If you don't want to grow your own, don't worry. It has become a lot easier to find herbs in many green-groceries and supermarkets. If you can't get fresh herbs, just substitute dried.

You should have a few good vinegars and mustards. I often use balsamic vinegar to deglaze a pan, alternating with Champagne vinegar, rice wine vinegar, tarragon vinegar, or red wine vinegar. Some mustards I like are Malle strong Dijon, Colman's hot English, and green peppercorn. There are many other varieties, but I do not believe that artificially flavored vinegars and mustards should be the important taste carriers in a recipe. Use the best generic kinds of each and build upon the other ingredients to get your flavor.

Grains give dishes texture and body and they help to fill you up. Try quinoa, a phenomenal grain that is high in protein. It is very easy to prepare using the instructions on the package and you can serve it in place of rice or potatoes with any recipe that calls for either. I don't give you any recipes specifically requiring quinoa, but I suggest it as an alternate. Wehani rice is only one of several new varieties of brown rice you can try. It is chewy and flavorful, not at all like the old-fashioned white rice you grew up with. I buy wehani in my local supermarket. It is a dark red, longer grained rice that is really good and easy to prepare. Your neighborhood health food store will surely carry it; if not, ask them to order it. It is grown in California and is well worth finding.

Stock up on all kinds of interesting pasta when you go on this program—I rely on pasta for many of my meals. I prefer dried to fresh; I think it tastes better, and you can't ruin it by overcooking as easily as you can the fresh pasta. Make sure that the pasta doesn't contain eggs—the only thing good pasta should contain is flour and water. I also prefer whole-wheat pasta because it has a "meaty" flavor and it gives you something to chew on—it bites back. The shape and size of pasta you choose to eat is totally up to you. My recipe may call for linguine, but you are free to substitute penne or rigatoni or anything else you like.

I give you directions for preparing my "endless-variation pasta"—which is really any combination of vegetables, fish, seafood, or poultry, and pasta that you care to dream up. These directions will turn you into a creative pasta chef. I also include several specific pasta recipes that have proven very successful.

STAPLES

Having these staples on hand will help you to prepare the recipes in this book as well as your own variations.

anchovies
apple cider jelly (available in health-food stores, or see the recipe)
beans, canned (Goya) or dried
capers, brine packed
Cajun spice (Konriko)
cayenne pepper
clams, frozen
clam juice
flour, unbleached
fruit preserves, no sugar added (Smucker's, Polaner's, Sorrel Ridge)
garlic
herbs, fresh and dried
lentils (Legumor brand, green)
mustards: Malle Dijon, Colman's hot English, green peppercorn, white wine
oat bran
olive oil
olives
pasta, whole wheat and regular
peppercorns, black
quinoa
raisins
safflower oil
stocks: chicken and fish, homemade or commercial
Tabasco sauce
vegetables, fresh and frozen
vegetables, root: onions, potatoes
vinegars: balsamic, Champagne, red wine, rice wine, tarragon
walnuts
white wine

EQUIPMENT

Although it seems to me that I cook many of my recipes in one sauté pan, here is a list of some additional equipment you may want to have on hand. You can be creative in your use of substitutes. (See the section on stocks for the equipment needed in stock preparation.)

a good, sharp chef's knife 10 to 12 inches long
a paring knife
large chef's spoons
a chef's fork
spatulas: wood (for scraping nonstick pans) and metal
a chopping board
sauté pans, 8, 10, and 12 inch
a large pasta pot, about ten quarts
a large strainer
several heavy-bottomed roasting pans of different sizes
a black cast-iron 9-inch skillet
a wok lid
nonstick 10- and 8-inch baking pans
a nonstick 10-inch pie pan
nonstick cookie sheets
muffin tins
foil muffin cups
mixing bowls
a grill
fruitwood and charcoal for grilling
a food processor

Of course you need some kind of stove, oven, and broiler. Everyone's oven isn't calibrated equally, but oven temperature really doesn't make a difference with this kind of food. For most of my roasting recipes I turn up the oven to its highest setting. This is the way food is cooked in restaurants.

METHODS

It will be helpful for you to understand some very simple cooking skills as they apply to the foods you will prepare on this program.

SEARING

When you sear fish or shrimp or any other food, heat a pan until it is very hot. Don't add oil. Put the food into the hot pan—it will smoke and get brown and somewhat burned on the outside. Sear it for only a few minutes on each side, so that the inside remains soft and moist.

If you rub the fish or other food with Cajun spices and sear it in a very small quantity of oil, you will have a "blackened" dish.

SAUTÉING

Sautéing food means cooking it in a pan over medium to high heat in a little fat. When you sauté, you brown the food on one side, turn it, and brown it on the other side.

SWEATING

When you sweat food, you cook it in a small amount of oil over low heat, covered. Sweated onions don't become brown, they become translucent.

GRILLING

Grilling over a charcoal or wood fire is a good, low-fat method of cooking, and I love the extra flavor imparted by the "burn" it puts on food. My only complaint is that when you grill chicken or fish, the tasty, fragrant juices drip into the fire. Roasting allows you to save those juices in the pan.

When you grill small birds, use the method I outline in my recipe for Grilled Baby Chicken (Poussin) Stuffed with Sage. Use a chef's fork to turn the bird every 3 to 5 minutes, making sure every bit of skin is cooked to a golden brown. When all the skin is browned, the bird will be completely cooked.

ROASTING

In the recipes that follow, I give directions to roast chicken at high oven temperatures so that the skin becomes crisp and golden brown. Turn the food you are roasting so that every part is exposed to heat, and never cover it. Roasting food ensures delicious pan juices and those crunchy burnt-on particles of food that enrich a sauce.

DEGLAZING

In low-fat cooking there will be little morsels of browned or burnt food sticking to the bottom of the pan. These add a great deal of flavor to the dish when you deglaze the pan, as follows. Add wine, vinegar, or stock (or any combination of the three) to the pan and move it around over medium heat, scraping particles off the bottom with a spatula. You will dislodge more cooked-on particles if you use a stainless steel or black iron pan, rather than a nonstick pan. You can deglaze a pan after the large pieces of food are removed, or you can leave the food in.

The principle is the same for deglazing in a roasting pan as it is for a sauté pan. After you have roasted a chicken and you have burnt particles stuck to the bottom of the roasting pan, tilt the pan so that the fat rises to the top. Pour off the chicken fat and keep all the good chicken juices. Then put the roasting pan on top of the stove, add stock or vinegar or white wine, turn up the heat to medium, and start scraping. Get all the crunchy bits off the bottom of the pan and use them in your sauce.

REDUCING A SAUCE

It is only common sense that the more you reduce or concentrate a sauce, the more flavorful it will become. After deglazing a pan I often cook down the liquid until it is thick and syrupy enough to coat a spoon lightly. I then brush the flavorful sauce on top of the food or put it underneath the food that I am serving. There is no perfect cooking time for reducing a sauce. *Constantly taste it as it reduces*, dipping in either a spoon or your fingertip, to test the level of concentration. Chefs call this process tasting "on the way down."

None of my recipes specifically calls for reductions of stock, but these are easily prepared and can add a lot of flavor to a dish. For directions, see the individual stock recipes in this chapter.

BUILDING A SAUCE

In my former life, I almost always finished off the perfect sauce with butter and cream. Clearly, I can't cook that way anymore. Therefore, over the last couple of years I have developed a system whereby I get all of the intense flavor of the cooking juices and the deglazing liquid with none of the fat.

Once you get a critical mass of liquid in a pan and start to reduce it, all the flavors—including the scrapings, stock, wine, vinegar, spices—will concentrate and intensify. Adding back ingredients and cooking further "builds" the sauce.

Here is the method: After you have deglazed the sauté pan or roasting pan and reduced the sauce, add more stock, wine, and/or vinegar in any proportions. You may add a few tablespoons of a stock reduction here, as well (see Stocks and Reductions). As you add, continue cooking down the sauce. As with reductions, *keep tasting* until you reach the point of flavor and concentration you want.

MARINATING

When you marinate a chicken or a piece of fish, you are using oil as a vehicle to impregnate the flesh **with the flavor of herbs**, spices, and garlic. As the food marinates, move it around in the oil—it doesn't have to be covered by the marinade. After the food has been marinated, place it on a rack and let all the marinade drip off. Refrigerate the mixture and save it for the next time; it will keep for up to one month.

You can also use an oil-free marinade like soy sauce or lime juice. This doesn't stick to the meat as well as the oil does, therefore it doesn't add as much flavor.

THE RECIPES

This list of dishes is not divided into appetizers and main courses because most of the dishes will do equally well in either category. White Bean Soup can be a complete meal or an appetizer; so can White-Clam Pizza or Linguine with Garlic and Anchovies.

Try the oat-bran muffins for breakfast or with any meal, and the oat-bran cookies as a snack or dessert. And my fruit creations are good for dessert, snacks, or celebrations.

STOCKS AND REDUCTIONS
Fish Stock and Reduction
Chicken Stock and Reduction

SOUPS
White Bean Soup
Black Bean Soup
Wild Mushroom Soup
Hearty Turkey and Potato Soup

The Recipes

SALADS
Watercress and Endive Salad with Walnuts and Parmesan Cheese
Lobster or Shrimp Salad
Roasted Chicken Salad
Chunky Tuna Salad
No-Oil Vinaigrette

PASTA
David's Endless-Variation Pasta
Whole-Wheat Pasta Elbows with Shrimp, Crab, Black Beans, and Peas
Whole-Wheat Pasta with Tomatoes, Capers, and Onions
Pasta with Grilled Shrimp, Leeks, and Shiitake Mushrooms
Linguine with Garlic and Anchovies

PIZZA
David's French Bread Pizza Dough
White-Clam Pizza
Cheeseless Wild Mushroom and Black Olive Pizza

FISH AND SHELLFISH
Spicy Swordfish, Grilled or Seared
Grilled or Broiled Swordfish on Melted Leeks
Seared Tuna with Mustard and Onions
Grilled or Seared Shrimp with Steamed Broccoli
Grilled or Seared Shrimp with Black Bean Sauce
Mussels, Shallots, and Coriander in Spicy Broth
Roasted Lobster with Tarragon
Crispy Scallops with Mushrooms on Spicy Rice

POULTRY
Roast Chicken Chez Louis
Chicken Roasted on Potato Slices, Tomato Slices, and Mashed Garlic
Roast Chicken Stuffed with Grilled Shiitake Mushrooms and Deglazed with Balsamic Vinegar

Grilled Baby Chicken (Poussin) Stuffed with Sage
Tasty Grilled Quail
Turkey and/or Chicken Burgers
Baked Potato Skin with Grilled Turkey and Onions

VEGETABLES
Potato Pie Chez Louis
Potato Pie with Clams and Coriander
Roasted Mushrooms and Garlic Chez Louis
Roasted Vegetables
Baked Potato with Salsa and Seared Shrimp
Killer Potatoes with Hot Chilies
Chinese Garlic Broccoli
Steamed Cabbage with Chinese Black Beans
Crusty Brown Rice with Vegetables
Lentils with Vegetables

CONDIMENTS
Tapenade
Apple Cider Jelly

FRUIT
Apples Baked with Apple Cider Jelly and Cinnamon
Fruit Floating in Fruit
No-Cholesterol Strawberry Tart/Pie

SNACKS AND FALLBACKS
Spicy Popcorn
Potato Crisps

MUFFINS AND COOKIES
David's Oat-Bran Muffins
David's Oat-Bran Cookies

The Recipes

STOCKS AND REDUCTIONS

The following recipes for chicken stock and fish stock are as good and comprehensive as any you will find. I perfected them with Michèle Urvater, with whom I wrote *Cooking the Nouvelle Cuisine in America,* and they appeared in that book substantially as you see them here. They are much more detailed than any of the recipes that follow them, and the careful instructions help you to produce excellent results. These stocks will add wonderful flavor and dimension to your cooking.

If you don't want to make your own stocks, you can use any of several good commercial brands; for fish stock, you can often substitute bottled clam juice, but bear in mind that the juice sometimes can be saltier than stock.

The theory behind making a stock and reducing it to a sticky, viscous consistency is that reduction concentrates and intensifies the flavors in the stock. Although none of the recipes I give you in this book calls for reductions as such, one of the secrets of great cooking is adding a few tablespoons of a reduction to a dish to kick up its flavor.

Take the extra time to make the chicken stock reduction, store it in your freezer in an ice-cube tray, and try adding it to any of the chicken recipes in this book that calls for a sauce. You won't be disappointed.

The bonus you get in every reduction is enhanced flavor with negligible extra calories, no fat, and very little cholesterol.

FISH STOCK AND REDUCTION

■   ■   ■

To prepare this recipe, you will need a 10- to 12-quart stockpot, cheesecloth, a strainer or a sieve, and a skimmer or shallow spoon.

7 pounds roughly chopped flat fish carcasses (bones and heads), such as sole or flounder, with gills removed
2 pounds onions, peeled and quartered
6–8 sprigs Italian parsley, stems removed
2 cups dry white wine
1 bay leaf
14–18 whole black peppercorns

■

1   Place all the ingredients in the stockpot and fill it with water to a point two inches from the top of the pot.
2   Bring all the ingredients to a slow boil over medium heat. As the water begins to boil, a grayish scum will rise to the surface. Lower the heat to ensure that the scum does not rise over the edge of the pot. Remove the scum with a large, shallow spoon. Do not be afraid to scoop out all traces of the scum and lose

The Recipes

some of the surrounding stock. You can always replace the liquid with fresh water.

3. When the water is about to boil again, reduce the heat and simmer the stock slowly for 30 minutes, skimming and replacing the scum with fresh water every 10 minutes. The stock is properly simmering when there is movement on the surface of the water in the form of tiny bubbles. If the bubbles get too large, the stock is boiling; you must reduce the heat.

4. After the stock has simmered for 30 minutes, turn off the heat. Strain all the stock through a cheesecloth-lined sieve into another stockpot or large container. You can accomplish this in one of two ways. If you are strong, simply pour the stock through the cheesecloth from one pot to the next. Then discard the cooked solids. However, a safer technique is to use a large ladle and transfer the stock through the cheesecloth in smaller amounts. When most of the liquid has been removed, scoop out the remaining solids and discard them, using a skimmer or slotted spoon. Remove only the solids; don't lose any of the stock in the process. Make sure the discarded solids are disposed of in a waterproof container because they are messy.

5. Once the solids are removed, pour the remaining stock through the cheesecloth into the other stockpot or container.

6. At this point the basic fish stock is ready to be used or stored in the refrigerator overnight. If you are storing the stock, cool it first, uncovered, to room temperature and then refrigerate it, covered. The next day remove any additional scum that has congealed on the surface. Fish stock will last only two days in the refrigerator; it freezes very well, however.

7. If you intend to continue cooking the stock down to a reduction, return the stock to a stockpot and place it back on the heat. As the stock begins to boil, it will throw off more grayish scum. Keep removing the scum with a large, shallow spoon until the stock can be brought to a rolling boil without foaming over the top of the pot.

8. Depending on the size of your stockpot, the liquid should boil down to about 1 pint in 2 to 4 hours. (The wider the base of the stockpot, the faster the stock will reduce.) When there is about 1 pint of liquid remaining in the pot, remove the reduction. Make sure you scrape all of it from the sides and bottom of the pot. Store the reduction, covered, in a plastic container or in foil-covered ice-cube trays, in which the reduction may be easily frozen. The reduction will keep in a covered container in the refrigerator for a week to ten days.

■ MAKES 4–5 QUARTS OF FISH STOCK OR 1 PINT OF REDUCTION

CHICKEN STOCK AND REDUCTION

To prepare this recipe, you will need a large roasting pan, a 10- to 12-quart stockpot, cheesecloth, a strainer or a sieve, and a skimmer or a slotted spoon.

7 pounds of chicken carcasses, backs, and necks in any combination.
1 pound onions, peeled and roughly chopped into 1-inch pieces

The Recipes

1 pound carrots, scraped and roughly chopped into 1-inch pieces

1 leek, carefully washed and roughly chopped into 1-inch pieces (optional)

1 *bouquet garni* made up of:
- 6–8 sprigs parsley
- 1 bay leaf
- 14–18 whole black peppercorns
- 1 tablespoon fresh thyme or ¼ teaspoon dried
- 2 cloves garlic, unpeeled

■

1. Preheat the oven to 400°F.
2. Arrange all the chicken pieces in a roasting pan large enough to accommodate them in one layer. For best results, the pieces should be no larger than 2–3 inches.
3. Roast the bones in the oven for 1 hour. Remove the pan from the oven and toss the chopped vegetables on top of the bones. Add 2 cups water to the roasting pan and return it to the oven. Continue roasting for an additional ½ hour.
4. Transfer the contents of the roasting pan to a stockpot on top of the stove. Make sure you scrape out all the browned particles on the bottom of the pan into the stockpot. This will give your stock added flavor. (Note: The 2 cups of water were added to the roasting pan to make it easier to scrape the browned particles into the stockpot with the chicken and vegetables.)
5. Fill the stockpot with water to a point two inches from the top of the pot. (Note: It is not crucial that the amount of water added to the pot be exactly the same each time. You always are in complete control of the reduction because you can always reduce the stock to make it more intense and flavorful.)
6. Prepare the *bouquet garni* by enclosing all the ingredients in a piece of cheesecloth tied with a piece of string. Once this has

been completed, add the *bouquet garni* to the pot and make sure that it is completely submerged in the water.

7. Bring all the ingredients to a slow boil over medium heat in the stockpot. As the water begins to boil, the chicken fat will rise to the surface. Lower the heat to ensure that the fat does not rise over the edge. Remove the fat with a large, shallow spoon. Do not be afraid to scoop out all the traces of the fat and lose some of the surrounding stock. You can always replace the discarded liquid with fresh water.

8. When the stock is about to boil again, reduce the heat and simmer the stock for 3½ hours, skimming and replacing the fat with fresh water every hour. (Note: In the first hour you may have to skim the pot every 15 minutes or so.) The stock is properly simmering when there is movement on the surface of the water in the form of tiny bubbles. If the bubbles get too large, the stock is boiling; you must reduce the heat. As the stock simmers, the liquid will evaporate. Add water from time to time to maintain the contents of the pot at the same level.

9. After the stock has simmered for 3½ hours, turn off the heat. Strain all the stock through a cheesecloth-lined sieve into another stockpot or large container. You can accomplish this in one of two ways. If you are strong, simply pour the stock through a cheesecloth-lined sieve from one pot to the next. Then discard the cooked solids. However, a safer technique is to use a large ladle and transfer the stock through the cheesecloth in smaller amounts. When most of the liquid has been removed, scoop out the remaining solids and discard them, using a shallow spoon. Remove only the solids; don't lose any of the stock in the process. Make sure the discarded solids are disposed of in a waterproof container because they are messy.

10. Once all the chicken pieces and vegetables are removed, pour the remaining stock through the cheesecloth into the stockpot or container.

11. At this point the chicken stock is ready to be used or to be stored covered in the refrigerator overnight. In either case, you

The Recipes

must remove any additional fat that rises to the surface. If you leave the stock at this point and don't boil it down to reduction consistency, you must bring it back to a boil every third day in order to rid it of any potential bacteria that may accumulate. If you are storing the stock, cool it first, uncovered, to room temperature.

12 If you intend to reduce the stock, return it to a stockpot and place it back on the heat. As the stock begins to boil, it will throw off more fat. Keep removing the fat with a large, shallow spoon until the stock can be brought to a rolling boil without foaming over the top of the pot.

13 Depending on the size of your stockpot and the amount of stock you are making, the liquid should boil down to about 1 pint in 2 to 4 hours. The larger the surface area of the pot, the faster the stock will reduce. When there is about 1 pint of liquid remaining in the pot (measure if you're not sure), remove the reduction from the sides and bottom of the pot. Let the liquid cool, uncovered, in the refrigerator, then store the reduction, covered, in a plastic container or in foil-covered ice-cube trays in which the reduction may be easily frozen.

■ MAKES 4–5 QUARTS OF CHICKEN STOCK OR 1 PINT OF REDUCTION

SOUPS

WHITE BEAN SOUP

■ ■ ■

It is a good idea to double or triple this recipe so that you can have a large batch of soup to keep in the refrigerator or freezer. A filling soup is one dish I can always rely on if I want to eat dinner before I go out to dinner (see strategies, chapter 8).

2 tablespoons olive oil
½ cup minced leeks, the white and tender green parts only
½ cup minced onions
2 tablespoons chopped shallots
¼ cup Champagne vinegar
½ cup white wine
4 cups chicken stock
2 cups cooked white beans prepared from dry beans, or 1 can white beans (16 ounces), rinsed well and drained
salt and pepper to taste
4 tablespoons chopped coriander or Italian parsley

1. If you are using dried beans, prepare them according to the directions on the package. Set them aside.
2. Heat the olive oil in a sauté pan. Add the leeks and sauté for 15 minutes over low heat. Add the onions and sauté for an additional 10 minutes. Add the shallots and sauté 5 minutes more. At this point, all the vegetables should be translucent.
3. Turn up the heat to medium, add the vinegar and white wine, and deglaze the pan.
4. Pour the chicken stock into a pot large enough to hold all the ingredients comfortably. Add the vegetables and the cooked or canned beans and heat to a simmer. Cook the soup over low heat for 30 minutes. Season to taste with salt and pepper. Garnish each portion with chopped coriander or Italian parsley.

■ MAKES 4 SERVINGS

BLACK BEAN SOUP

■   ■   ■

This is a heartier, spicier soup than the delicate white bean soup. On a cold winter day it makes a perfect meal with a chunk of crusty French bread. (Be sure to throw away the middle of the bread and eat just the crust.)

2 cups cooked black beans prepared from dry beans, or 1 can black beans (16 ounces), rinsed well and drained

2 tablespoons olive oil
½ cup minced leeks, the white and tender green parts only
1 cup minced carrots
½ cup minced celery
½ cup minced onions
4 cloves garlic, peeled and mashed
2 tablespoons chopped shallots
¼ cup Champagne vinegar
½ cup white wine
4 cups chicken stock
salt and cayenne pepper to taste
4 tablespoons chopped coriander or Italian parsley

■

1. If you are using dried beans, prepare them according to the directions on the package. Set them aside.
2. Heat the olive oil in a sauté pan. Add the leeks, carrots, and celery and sauté for 15 minutes over low heat. Add the onions and sauté an additional 10 minutes. Add the garlic and shallots and sauté 5 minutes more. At this point, all the vegetables should be translucent.
3. Add the vinegar and white wine, turn up the heat to medium, and deglaze the pan.
4. Place the chicken stock in a pot. Add the vegetables and cooked or canned beans to the stock and heat to a simmer. Cook the soup over low heat for 30 minutes. Season to taste with salt and cayenne pepper. Garnish each portion with chopped coriander or Italian parsley.

■ MAKES 4 SERVINGS

The Recipes

WILD MUSHROOM SOUP

■   ■   ■

This soup is especially delicious because you take the time to roast or grill the mushrooms before you add them to the chicken stock. You can use any kind of mushrooms for this soup, even domestic, but the meatier and tastier the mushrooms, the more flavorful the soup.

1 pound shiitake mushrooms, or any other kind of mushrooms you choose, cleaned and stemmed (about 4 cups)
2 tablespoons olive oil, plus olive oil for brushing the mushrooms
½ cup diced onions
½ cup diced carrots
2 tablespoons balsamic vinegar
4 cups chicken stock
1 cup white wine
salt, pepper, and Tabasco sauce to taste
2 tablespoons chopped coriander or Italian parsley

■

1. If you are grilling the mushrooms, prepare a charcoal or wood fire. If you are roasting them, preheat the oven to its highest setting.
2. Brush the mushrooms lightly with olive oil. Grill them 4 minutes on each side or roast them for 12 minutes. Set them aside.

3. Heat the olive oil in a sauté pan and sauté the onions and carrots for about 5 minutes. Deglaze the pan with balsamic vinegar and set it aside.
4. Place the chicken stock and vegetables in a pot large enough to accommodate them comfortably and bring to a boil. Lower the heat, add the mushrooms, and stir well. Add the wine and continue to cook the soup down for 15 minutes. (The more you cook the soup and the more it reduces, the more concentrated the flavor.)
5. Season the soup to taste with the salt, pepper, and Tabasco. Garnish with coriander or Italian parsley.

■ MAKES 4 SERVINGS

HEARTY TURKEY AND POTATO SOUP

■   ■   ■

Fresh, sliced turkey meat has become available in most supermarkets, making a recipe like this one easy and quick to prepare. Turkey is a lean, excellent source of protein that adds flavor and texture to a soup. Add the turkey at the last moment so that it doesn't overcook and become tough.

2 cups chicken stock
½ pound (2 cups) boiling potatoes, peeled and cut into ½-inch chunks, about 2 cups chopped
½ cup chopped onions
½ cup chopped carrots
2 tablespoons balsamic vinegar
1 cup white wine
salt, pepper, and Tabasco sauce to taste
½ pound turkey scallops (about ¼-inch thick) cut into ¼-inch strips, about 1 cup
2 tablespoons chopped coriander or Italian parsley

■

1. Bring the stock to a boil in a pot large enough to hold all the ingredients. Lower the heat to a simmer; add the potatoes and cook 20 minutes.
2. While the potatoes are cooking, heat the olive oil in a sauté pan and sauté the onions and carrots 5 minutes. Deglaze the pan with balsamic vinegar and remove it from the heat.
3. Add the wine to the broth and potatoes. Add the onions and carrots. Cook an additional 10 minutes over medium heat. Add the turkey meat and cook 3 minutes or until the turkey is cooked through. Season the soup with salt, pepper, and Tabasco; remove from heat. Garnish with the coriander or Italian parsley.

■ MAKES 4 SERVINGS

SALADS

Watercress and Endive Salad with Walnuts and Parmesan Cheese

■   ■   ■

You may change the proportions of watercress and endive to suit your taste. Just be sure that the peppery watercress does not overpower the endive. You may also use any vinaigrette you choose for this salad, as long as it has a certain strength of flavor to stand up to the strongly flavored greens. The mustard in the vinaigrette below gives the dressing the kick it needs.

2 bunches watercress, washed and stemmed
4 medium-sized endives (more if you prefer)
¼ cup toasted walnuts, chopped coarsely
¼ cup grated parmesan cheese

1. Wash and dry the salad greens. Toss with the mustard vinaigrette (recipe follows).
2. Sprinkle the walnuts and cheese over the salad.

■ MAKES 4 SERVINGS

MUSTARD VINAIGRETTE

¼ teaspoon salt
¼ teaspoon pepper
1 teaspoon Dijon mustard
2 tablespoons red wine vinegar
3 tablespoons olive oil

Put all the ingredients in a small screw-top jar, cap the jar tightly, and shake it vigorously.

■ MAKES ¼ CUP VINAIGRETTE

LOBSTER OR SHRIMP SALAD

This salad is a treat served for lunch or dinner, and it is a natural for preparing at home and carrying to work. Served on pita bread, it makes an easy, convenient, and elegant sandwich.

4 medium tomatoes
2 tablespoons chopped shallots
1 cup chopped celery
¼ cup pitted Niçoise olives
1 tablespoon chopped fresh tarragon or ½ teaspoon dried
1 pound cooked lobster meat or cooked shrimp, shelled and deveined
5 tablespoons No-Oil Vinaigrette (see recipe, page 192)
salt and pepper to taste

■

1. Chop the tomatoes into ½-inch chunks. Combine them in a bowl with the shallots, celery, olives, and tarragon.
2. Add the lobster meat or shrimp and combine well. Mix in the vinaigrette, taste, and season with salt and pepper. Serve the salad on a bed of lettuce or use it as the filling for sandwiches.

■ MAKES 4 INDIVIDUAL SALADS OR SANDWICHES

The Recipes

ROASTED CHICKEN SALAD

■ ■ ■

The pieces of roasted chicken meat should be left as large as possible. This salad has a certain trencherman's quality—it is the kind of food you want to eat with your hands, along with a crusty loaf of French or Italian bread.

I can't really call this a quick recipe because the first step is roasting a chicken. But the next time you prepare Roasted Chicken Chez Louis, cook two chickens and reserve one for this dish. If you are roasting a chicken especially for salad you can skip searing the skin if you like, although the skin is included in the salad and searing adds an extra touch.

Meat of one 2½- to 3-pound roasted chicken, removed from the bone (see recipe for Roasted Chicken Chez Louis)
½ pound (about 8) small new potatoes or regular boiling potatoes (about 4 medium)
½ cup pitted Niçoise olives
½ cup diced green or red pepper
6–8 tablespoons No-Oil Vinaigrette (see recipe, page 192)
salt and pepper to taste
8 large leaves romaine lettuce

1. Roast the chicken. Remove the meat from the bones, keeping it in large chunks with the skin on. Set aside the chicken meat.
2. If the potatoes are very small, leave them whole. If not, cut them into ¼-inch slices. Bring a large pot of water to a boil and add the potatoes. Boil them until a skewer piercing them comes out clean.
3. Combine the chicken, potatoes, olives, peppers, and vinaigrette in a bowl. Season the salad with salt and pepper. Arrange the romaine leaves on a serving plate and pile the chicken salad on top. Serve the salad cold, warm, or hot.

■ MAKES 4–6 SERVINGS

CHUNKY TUNA SALAD

This is a special tuna salad prepared with freshly grilled or seared tuna. Of course, if time is short you can substitute canned tuna, but I believe that fresh tastes better. The salad may be served cold or at room temperature.

½ pound (about 8) small new potatoes or regular boiling potatoes (about 4 medium)

1 pound tuna steak about 1 inch thick
4 medium tomatoes, cut into 1-inch chunks
¼ cup pitted Niçoise olives
¼ cup minced onions
¼ cup thinly sliced scallions, white and tender green parts only
¼ cup roughly chopped radishes
1 small tin anchovies, drained of oil and chopped into ¼-inch pieces
6–8 tablespoons No-Oil Vinaigrette (see recipe, page 192)
salt and pepper to taste
8 leaves romaine lettuce

■

1. If you are going to grill the tuna, prepare a wood or charcoal fire.
2. If the potatoes are small, leave them whole. If not, cut them into ¼-inch slices. Bring a large pot of water to a boil and add the potatoes. Boil them until a skewer piercing them comes out clean. Drain the potatoes and set aside.
3. Grill the tuna or sear it in a hot pan 3 to 5 minutes on each side. Cut the tuna into 1-inch chunks.
4. Combine the olives, onions, radishes, anchovies, and vinaigrette in a large bowl. Mix them together very well.
5. Add the tuna, potatoes, and tomatoes, and mix together gently. Season with salt and pepper. Serve the salad on a bed of romaine lettuce leaves.

■ MAKES 4 SERVINGS

No-Oil Vinaigrette

■   ■   ■

This vinaigrette is quick to prepare, as well as tasty. And it keeps in the refrigerator—just shake it well before you use it. You can vary the taste by using different vinegars and by using any fresh or dried herbs, and you can combine herbs if you choose. Best of all, this dressing contains no fat.

1 cup white wine
½ cup of your favorite vinegar
3 tablespoons strong Dijon mustard (I like Malle)
1 tablespoon chopped fresh sage or ½ teaspoon dried
1 tablespoon chopped shallots
salt and pepper to taste

■

In no particular order, add all the ingredients to a screw-top jar. Close the jar tightly, shake it well, and serve the vinaigrette over your favorite salad.

■   MAKES 1½ CUPS

The Recipes

PASTA

DAVID'S ENDLESS-VARIATION PASTA

▪ ▪ ▪

This is the completely adaptable, the bottomless, the endless-variation pasta recipe. Actually it is not a recipe for, but a theory of, pasta. Using it you can take any number of different ingredients and combine them into creative pasta dishes. Simply ask yourself: "What do I want to eat today, and can it be combined with pasta?"

If you like onions and you like Brussels sprouts and you like shrimp—combine them, perhaps with whole-wheat spaghetti. If you like melted leeks and chicken—combine them with penne or linguine. If you like garlic, tomatoes, and chickpeas, or you like onions, tomatoes, and olives—combine them with any pasta you feel like eating.

Build your pasta creation. The basic ingredient categories are

pasta
oil
onions (that is, onions, shallots, and garlic)
vegetables
fish, shellfish, or fowl
flavorings (salt, pepper, herbs, wine, and vinegar)

■

You aren't restricted to one from each category and you can skip categories. Your dish can contain several vegetables and no fish or fowl. You can skip the wine, vinegar, and even the salt and pepper. But you really should base your sauce on sautéd or sweated onions of some kind.

The basic steps are: *choice, preparation, cooking, and combination*. The whole creative process takes only minutes and the result will be exactly to your taste.

1. CHOICE

First choose your pasta, whole wheat or regular, dried or fresh (but made without eggs), in any shape or size. Fettuccine, angel hair, spaghetti, macaroni, pappardelle, and linguine are only a few of the many choices. Allow about ¼ pound of pasta per serving.

Set aside your two tablespoons of oil—my choice is olive oil. It will be used to cover the bottom of a sauté pan and to cook all your ingredients.

Choose onions, garlic, or shallots. The amount and combination is entirely up to you. I almost always begin my pasta recipes with onions and build from there.

Choose the vegetables you want to eat from anything on the Yes list of vegetables. How about cabbage, cauliflower, peas, zucchini, tomatoes, or mushrooms? Or you may use melted leeks or cooked white beans that you prepared earlier or reserved from another recipe. Again, the amount is up to you. You can prepare any of the vegetables ahead of time and reheat them when you combine your ingredients.

If you want to add fish, shellfish, or fowl to your dish, consult the Yes list of foods and choose salmon, swordfish, shrimp, turkey, or anything that appeals to you in amounts of your choice.

2. PREPARATION

Bring a large pot of lightly salted water to a boil. Add the pasta and cook until it is done to your taste.

While the pasta is cooking, peel and slice your onions (shallots, garlic). Clean and slice your vegetables if necessary. Cut the fish or poultry into small, regular pieces so that it can be cooked quickly.

3. COOKING

Heat the oil in a large sauté pan. Sauté or sweat the onions (and/or garlic and shallots) until they soften.

Add the vegetables and cover the pan. Steam the vegetables with the onion mixture until they are crisp but tender.

Add the vinegar or wine.

Remove the vegetables and keep them warm. Add the fish, shellfish, or fowl to the hot pan and sear it quickly on both sides.

Return the vegetables and onions to the pan and season to taste.

Keep the mixture warm.

By now the pasta should be cooked. Drain it and combine it with the vegetable mixture.

Presto! You have created a pasta dish!

Whole-Wheat Pasta Elbows with Shrimp, Crab, Black Beans, and Peas

■   ■   ■

The key to the success of this dish is not to overcook the shrimp and the crab. The black-bean mixture can be prepared ahead of time and combined with the just-cooked seafood at the last minute.

1 pound whole-wheat pasta elbows
2 tablespoons olive oil
½ cup chopped onions
2 cloves garlic, peeled and mashed
8 ounces canned black beans, rinsed and drained, or 1 cup cooked black beans prepared from dry beans
1 cup white wine
¼ cup red wine vinegar
salt and pepper to taste
½ pound shrimp, cleaned and deveined
½ pound fresh lump crabmeat, picked over
1 cup fresh or frozen green peas

The Recipes

1. Bring a large pot of salted water to a boil. Cook the pasta until it is al dente. Drain and set aside.
2. Heat the olive oil in a sauté pan. Sauté the onions and garlic for 5 minutes or until lightly browned.
3. Add the black beans and the wine to the sauté pan and cook for 2 to 3 minutes or until they are heated through. Deglaze the pan with the vinegar and set it aside.
4. In a separate pan, barely cook the shrimp and crabmeat over medium heat, about 1 minute on each side for the shrimp.
5. Return the pan of black beans to medium heat. Add the peas and cook for 2 minutes, then add the shrimp and crabmeat. Cook until the shrimp and crabmeat are heated through. Season with salt and pepper.
6. Place the mixture in a large serving bowl and add the pasta elbows. Combine well.

■ MAKES 4 SERVINGS

WHOLE-WHEAT PASTA WITH TOMATOES, CAPERS, AND ONIONS

This is basically a pasta primavera—a pasta with a chunky vegetable sauce. Use the vegetables as called for below or use any substitutes that appeal to you; change the proportions too, if you like. Served at room temperature, this makes a delicious and attractive buffet dish.

2 tablespoons olive oil
½ cup chopped onions
2 tablespoons chopped shallots
2 cups chopped tomatoes, fresh or canned
4 tablespoons brine-packed capers, drained
¼ cup balsamic vinegar
½ cup white wine
1 pound whole-wheat pasta
salt and pepper to taste
4 tablespoons chopped coriander

1. Bring a large pot of salted water to a boil.
2. While the water is heating, heat the olive oil in a sauté pan. Sauté the onions and shallots in the oil until the onions are translucent. Add the tomatoes and the capers, sauté for 5 minutes over medium heat, and then add the vinegar and the wine.
3. Cook, stirring, for an additional 15 to 20 minutes until the sauce begins to thicken.
4. While the sauce is cooking, boil the pasta until it reaches the al dente stage, about 7 to 9 minutes. Remove the pot from the heat, drain the pasta, and transfer it to a large serving bowl.
5. Season the sauce with salt and pepper, pour it on top of the pasta, and mix thoroughly. Sprinkle the coriander on top of the pasta and serve. The pasta is good served hot or at room temperature.

■ MAKES 4 SERVINGS

Pasta with Grilled Shrimp, Leeks, and Shiitake Mushrooms

■ ■ ■

This is one of my more time-consuming pasta recipes because it requires melted leeks. You may want to prepare them in advance, as I suggest in the recipe for Grilled Swordfish on Melted Leeks. With the prepared leeks on hand, you can throw this pasta together in minutes.

½ pound melted leeks (see pages 210–211)
1 tablespoon olive oil
1 pound pasta, any kind
5 cloves garlic, peeled and mashed
½ pound shiitake mushrooms, cleaned and stems removed
1 pound shrimp, shelled and deveined
½ cup Champagne vinegar
1 cup white wine
salt and pepper to taste
4 tablespoons chopped Italian parsley

■

1. Reheat the melted leeks if necessary.
2. Bring a large pot of salted water to a boil. Add the pasta and cook until al dente, about 7 to 9 minutes.
3. Coat a nonstick pan with the olive oil. Sauté the garlic over low heat for 2 minutes. Add the mushrooms, toss them around, and then add the shrimp. Cook the mixture 3 minutes and then remove the shrimp, mushrooms, and garlic from the pan. The shrimp will be undercooked, but they will finish cooking later.
4. Pour the vinegar and wine into the pan and add the reserved leeks. Cook for 3 to 4 minutes, add the shrimp mixture, and season with salt and pepper. Keep everything warm over low heat.
5. Drain the pasta and place it in a large serving bowl. Add the shrimp mixture and combine well. Serve in individual bowls garnished with parsley.

■ MAKES 4 SERVINGS

LINGUINE WITH GARLIC AND ANCHOVIES

This is meant to be a "dry" pasta; the sauce mixture will barely coat the noodles. The coriander gives the dish a fresh-from-the-garden taste.

Although I give directions to salt the pasta to taste, it is not likely that you will need additional salt, given the anchovies in the sauce.

2 tablespoons olive oil
6 cloves garlic, peeled and mashed
½ cup minced onions
2 tablespoons capers in brine, drained
1 pound linguine
4 tablespoons chopped anchovies
salt, pepper, and Tabasco sauce to taste
4 tablespoons chopped coriander

■

1. Bring a large pot of salted water to a boil.
2. While the water is heating, heat the olive oil in a sauté pan. Combine the garlic, onions, and capers and sweat them. When done, the onions should be barely translucent. Remove the pan from the heat.
3. Add the linguine to the boiling water and cook until al dente, about 7 to 9 minutes.
4. Put the sauté pan back over a low flame and add the anchovies to the vegetable mixture, stirring constantly.
5. When the pasta is done, drain it and transfer it to a serving bowl. Add the anchovy mixture and season to taste with salt, pepper, and Tabasco. Using two large chef's spoons, stir and toss the linguine vigorously. Sprinkle the coriander on top and serve immediately.

■ MAKES 4 SERVINGS

The Recipes

PIZZA

DAVID'S FRENCH BREAD PIZZA DOUGH

■   ■   ■

The finest pizza crust you can make is this one, based on the recipe for my French bread. It will be crisp, yeasty, fragrant, and delicious—the perfect vehicle for my fat-free white-clam or fresh vegetable pizzas, and for your own imaginative turns on these recipes.

The recipe will make six pizza shells approximately 16 inches in diameter and will keep in the refrigerator for a week to ten days. Don't cut the recipe in half! This recipe will not work properly with any lesser amounts of ingredients. After you have made one or two pies, the original pies for which you mixed this batch of pizza dough, you may be surprised to see that the extra dough you have sitting in the refrigerator will become your inspiration. You will want to invent your own recipes or to lighten some of your old favorites. You will see how far an excellent crust can take a pizza.

2⅔ cups warm water (approximately 90° to 100°F)
1½ ounces cake yeast or 2 packages granular yeast
6 cups unbleached all-purpose flour, plus approximately 1 cup extra for kneading
4 teaspoons salt

■

1. Put ⅔ cup of warm water in a measuring cup. Add the yeast and stir until the yeast dissolves.
2. Put 6 cups of flour and the salt in the bowl of an electric mixer equipped with a dough hook.
3. Add 2 cups of warm water and the yeast mixture to the flour. Mix on low speed for one minute.
4. Lift the dough hook. This is a damp dough. The object of this recipe is to use as little flour as possible. You should not need more than the six original cups and the one additional cup. If the dough seems too damp, however, add about ¼ cup more flour. If it seems a little dry, add up to ¼ cup more water. In any case, let the dough stand without stirring or mixing for two minutes.
5. Beat again on medium speed for 3 minutes.
6. Let the dough rest for 1 minute.
7. Beat on medium speed for 1 minute.
8. Let the dough rest for 1 minute.
9. Beat a final time for 1 minute. The dough will be fairly sticky.
10. Generously flour a flat, cool surface, preferably marble, using the flour from the additional cup. Scrape the dough out onto the floured surface. Using a pastry scraper, scrape the dough from the sides to the middle. Sprinkle the top of the dough with flour. Flour your fingers and knead the dough about 5 to 10 seconds. Shape it into a light, loose, nonsticky ball.
11. Drop the dough into a floured bowl. Cover with plastic wrap.
12. Put the bowl into a warm place—a gas oven with the pilot light on and the door ajar; a closet, wrapped in a blanket or towel—

The Recipes

and let it rise until doubled in bulk. This should take about 1½ hours. Or, put the dough in a refrigerator, where it should double in about 12 hours.

13. Generously flour a flat surface and turn and scrape the dough out onto it. If the dough is stuck in the bowl, scrape out as much as you can. Clean and dry the bowl and sprinkle it with 2 teaspoons of flour.

14. Scrape the dough from the sides to the middle on the floured surface until it can be shaped into a nonsticky ball. Keep the surface and your hands floured as you work. Shape the dough into a ball and drop it into the clean, floured bowl. Sprinkle with a little flour from the additional cup. Cover and return to a warm place to rise until doubled in bulk.

15. Repeat steps 13 and 14.

16. Scrape the dough out of the bowl onto a floured surface and divide it into 6 portions. Shape each into a ball and let it rise at room temperature on the floured surface for 15 to 20 minutes so that the gluten in the dough relaxes. Following the instructions for White-Clam Pizza, shape as many pizza crusts as you will be using, one crust from each ball of dough. Refrigerate any leftover dough, well wrapped in plastic wrap, for a week to ten days.

■ MAKES 6 PIZZA SHELLS, EACH APPROXIMATELY 16 INCHES IN DIAMETER

WHITE-CLAM PIZZA

■   ■   ■

The longer I have been on my program, the more I have come to appreciate crisp, low-fat pizzas that are sprinkled with only a small amount of grated cheese. (The optional grated parmesan cheese in this recipe contains less than 20 milligrams of cholesterol.) They can be prepared with any number of delicious toppings, and white-clam pizza represents the pinnacle of the art.

The pizza crust recipe I give you here is based on my French bread recipe. Preparing it will take some time, but the result is well worth it. You should try this recipe, if only for the experience of making and eating first-rate pizza dough.

If you prefer not to make your own bread dough for the crust, you can still enjoy fresh pizza. Spread the topping of your choice on pita bread, flatbread, French or Italian bread crusts, or even bagel crusts.

2 tablespoons olive oil
2 tablespoons white wine vinegar
8 ounces fresh, frozen, or canned clam meat
8 cloves garlic, peeled and mashed
salt and pepper to taste

½ pound bread dough (see recipe, pages 203–205) *or* 4 pita breads, cut in half horizontally, *or* a 16-inch piece of flatbread, *or* 1 small loaf of French or Italian bread, soft center removed, *or* 4 bagels, cut in half with centers removed.

¼ cup finely grated parmesan cheese, optional

■

1. Preheat the oven to its highest setting.
2. Combine the olive oil, vinegar, clams, and mashed garlic in a mixing bowl. Season with salt and pepper and set aside.
3. If you are using fresh dough, spread out the dough by pushing, pulling, and shaping until it is a very thin 16-inch disk. Transfer the dough to an ungreased nonstick pan, a pizza stone, or a round nonstick pizza pan. If you are not making your own dough, use one of the alternative crusts.
4. Spread the clam mixture over the surface of the crust. If you are using fresh dough, leave a 1-inch bare rim along the outside. If you are using an alternative crust, make the rim correspondingly smaller. If you like the outer crust very crisp, brush it lightly with olive oil. Sprinkle the entire pie with parmesan cheese if desired and bake for 7 to 9 minutes or until the clams are cooked. Serve immediately.

■ MAKES 1 16-INCH PIE, 8 PITA PIES, 1 16-INCH FLATBREAD PIE, OR 8 BAGEL PIES

Cheeseless Wild Mushroom and Black Olive Pizza

2 tablespoons olive oil
½ pound shiitake mushrooms, washed and stemmed
½ pound pitted Niçoise olives
3 tablespoons chopped shallots
3 tablespoons chopped chives

■

Heat the olive oil in a sauté pan and sauté the mushrooms, olives, and shallots for 5 minutes. Just before removing the pan from the heat, add the chopped chives and mix well. Spoon this topping over any of the prepared crusts listed in the recipe for White-Clam Pizza (see pages 206–207). Bake for 7 to 9 minutes.

FISH AND SHELLFISH

SPICY SWORDFISH, GRILLED OR SEARED

Swordfish is delicious and quick to prepare, and it marries well with interesting spices and seasonings. If you have sworn off red meat, chewy, hearty swordfish helps to bring back the memories.

For each portion:
1 tablespoon Cajun spice (Konrico)
1 swordfish steak
2 tablespoons balsamic vinegar, if you are searing fish
2 tablespoons chopped coriander or Italian parsley

1 If you are going to grill the fish, prepare a charcoal or wood fire.
2 Rub the Cajun spice onto both sides of the swordfish steak.
3 Grill the steak about 4 minutes on each side or until the fish is still moist in the center. Or, in a nonstick pan, sear each side

about 4 minutes or until the fish is still moist in the center. If you have seared the fish, remove it from the pan when done and then deglaze the pan with the balsamic vinegar.
4. Remove the swordfish steak to a dinner plate. If you have seared it, moisten it with the pan juices. Sprinkle it with coriander or Italian parsley and serve.

■ MAKES ONE SERVING

GRILLED OR BROILED SWORDFISH ON MELTED LEEKS

■   ■   ■

Melted leeks are one of the most delicious vegetables you can prepare. Since they take about a half hour to cook, it is a good idea to make them when you have time and store them in the refrigerator until you are ready to begin grilling or broiling. Then you can reheat them easily. The leeks go well with any kind of grilled fish or chicken.

2 pounds fresh leeks
2 tablespoons olive oil
salt and pepper to taste
¼ cup Champagne vinegar
1 pound swordfish steaks

■

1. Wash the leeks very carefully to make sure all the grit is removed. Cut off the brittle, stringy ends of the green stalks. Cut the white and tender green parts of the vegetable into strips approximately ½-inch thick by 4 inches long.
2. Heat the oil in a nonstick pan over high heat. Add the leeks and season with salt and pepper. Cover the pan to seal in the steam. If the leeks are piled high over the edge of the pan, use a wok lid or aluminum foil. Lower the heat and sweat the leeks until they are soft—"melted." This should take about 30 minutes. Just before removing the leeks, deglaze the pan with the Champagne vinegar.
3. Prepare a charcoal or wood fire or preheat a broiler.
4. Season the swordfish with salt and pepper. Grill the fish about 4 minutes on each side or broil until it is cooked through but still moist in the center. If you have refrigerated the cooked leeks, reheat them in a pan with ½ cup water. Spoon a portion of leeks on a dinner plate and place a swordfish steak over the leeks. Serve at once.

■ MAKES 2–3 SERVINGS

Seared Tuna with Mustard and Onions

Tuna is tasty and filling, and if you close your eyes you can even pretend that you are eating beef, because the tuna has a real "chew."

For each portion:
2 tablespoons Dijon mustard
salt and pepper to taste
1 tuna steak (whatever size you want to eat)
1 large onion, thinly sliced

1. Combine the mustard, salt, and pepper. Rub the mixture onto both sides of the tuna steak.
2. Cook the tuna over high heat in a nonstick pan to seal in its juices. A 1-inch-thick tuna steak will take 3 to 5 minutes on each side. Remove the tuna from the pan and set it aside.
3. Add the onions to the pan and sear 3 to 4 minutes. Deglaze the pan with the balsamic vinegar.
4. Place the tuna on a dinner plate and spoon the onion-vinegar mixture over it. Serve at once.

Note: You may want to add an additional tablespoon of mustard to the onions before serving.

■ MAKES 1 SERVING

GRILLED OR SEARED SHRIMP WITH STEAMED BROCCOLI

■   ■   ■

When you want to eat something tasty, simple, and elegant, this is the ideal recipe. Once the charcoal or wood fire is ready for grilling the shrimp, the actual cooking time is very short. But if you are hungry and you don't want to wait, sear the shrimp instead of grilling them. Then you will have this special dish on the table in minutes.

1 pound fresh broccoli, well washed
2 tablespoons olive oil
1 tablespoon puréed garlic
1 pound large shrimp, shelled and deveined
salt and pepper to taste

1. If you are grilling the shrimp, prepare a charcoal or wood fire.
2. Chop the broccoli into ½-inch cubes, or as close as you can get to cubes. Steam the broccoli in ½ inch of water in the bottom of a covered sauté pan 5 to 6 minutes or until it is crisp but tender.
3. Combine the oil and garlic. While the broccoli is steaming, rub the shrimp with the oil and garlic, salt, and pepper.
4. Either grill the shrimp or sear them in a nonstick pan for 2 to 3 minutes on each side. Set aside.
5. Drain the broccoli and divide it between two dinner plates. Arrange half the shrimp on top of each plate of broccoli. Serve immediately.

■ MAKES 4 SERVINGS

GRILLED OR SEARED SHRIMP WITH BLACK BEAN SAUCE

For an interesting variation, use ½ cup Chinese fermented black beans (available at Asian markets and some supermarkets) to replace ½ cup of the black beans.

2 cups cooked black beans prepared from dry beans, or one 16-ounce can black beans, rinsed well and drained
2 tablespoons olive oil
2 tablespoons minced shallots
½ cup chopped onions
1 cup chicken stock
¼ cup balsamic vinegar
salt and pepper to taste
3 tablespoons chopped parsley
1 pound large shrimp, shelled and deveined

1. If you are going to grill the shrimp, prepare a charcoal or wood fire.
2. If you are using dried beans, prepare them according to the directions on the package. Set them aside.
3. Heat the olive oil in a sauté pan. Sauté the shallots and onions with the beans over medium heat for 15 minutes.
4. Add the chicken stock to the mixture and bring it to a boil. Add the balsamic vinegar and cook down the mixture over high heat, stirring, until it is thick, approximately 15 minutes. Season the sauce with salt and pepper and set it aside.
5. Season the shrimp with pepper. Either grill the shrimp or sear them in a hot, ungreased or nonstick sauté pan for approximately 2 minutes on each side.
6. Reheat the black-bean sauce. Place the shrimp on a serving plate and spoon the black-bean sauce over them. Garnish with the chopped parsley. Serve immediately.

■ MAKES 4 SERVINGS

Mussels, Shallots, and Coriander in Spicy Broth

■ ■ ■

If you like bouillabaisse and fish stews, you really should try this recipe. Not only is it quick and delicious, it really fills you up. That is because the brown or wehani rice gives extra body to the dish.

4 cups fish stock
4 tablespoons minced shallots
¼ cup Champagne vinegar
2 pounds mussels, well scrubbed
2 cups cooked brown or wehani rice
salt and pepper to taste
¼ cup chopped coriander

■

1. Prepare your own fish stock (see recipe, page 174–175) or use a commercial alternative. Clam juice works well with this recipe.
2. Bring the stock to a boil and add the shallots and vinegar. Boil 1 minute. Add the mussels and steam them, covered, until the shells open, about 5 minutes. Discard any mussels that do not open.

3 Divide the cooked rice among 4 bowls or plates. Arrange a quarter of the mussels over the rice.
4 Season the stock with salt and pepper. Mix in the coriander and spoon the stock over the mussels. Serve immediately.

■. MAKES 4 SERVINGS

ROASTED LOBSTER WITH TARRAGON

■   ■   ■

This was the most popular way to prepare lobster when I was cooking at Restaurant Troisgros in France. On a typical day, it was the seafood entrée most in demand. The recipe calls for caramelized shallots, which are easily prepared.

For each portion:
2 tablespoons olive oil
2 tablespoons minced shallots
1 lobster (whatever size you want to eat)
1 tablespoon chopped fresh tarragon or ½ teaspoon dried
1 tablespoon Champagne vinegar
1 tablespoon minced Italian parsley
salt and pepper to taste

1. Preheat the oven to its highest setting.
2. Caramelize the shallots: Heat 1 tablespoon olive oil in a small nonstick sauté pan. Add the minced shallots and cook them over low heat until they are translucent and have begun to turn brown.
3. Split a live lobster in half by running a sharp knife through the back of the shell and pressing down.
4. Turn the lobster meat side up. Remove the intestinal sac near the head and discard it.
5. Mix together the shallots, tarragon, vinegar, olive oil, salt, and pepper in a small bowl. Spoon this mixture over the tail meat and cavity of the lobster.
6. Bake the lobster until tail meat is just cooked. This should take approximately 10 minutes for a 1½ pound lobster and 15 to 17 minutes for a 2–3 pound lobster. Sprinkle with the parsley and serve immediately.

■ MAKES 1 SERVING

The Recipes

CRISPY SCALLOPS WITH MUSHROOMS ON SPICY RICE

■   ■   ■

The scallops are "crispy" because they are seared over high heat for a short period of time. The Chinese black beans give the dish a certain Asian flair.

1 cup wehani rice (you can substitute another brown rice or quinoa)
2 tablespoons olive oil
½ cup minced onions
2 tablespoons minced shallots
2 tablespoons Chinese black beans (available in Asian markets and many supermarkets)
½ pound fresh mushrooms, cleaned, stemmed, and sliced into ¼-inch pieces. Domestic mushrooms work well in this dish.
¼ cup rice wine vinegar
salt and pepper to taste
1 pound sea scallops or bay scallops
3 tablespoons chopped Italian parsley

1. Prepare the rice according to package directions and set it aside.
2. Heat the olive oil in a sauté pan. Sauté the onions, shallots, black beans, and mushrooms for 5 minutes over medium heat until lightly browned. Deglaze the pan with the vinegar.
3. Season the scallops and sear them in a very hot sauté pan for 2 minutes on each side. Remove the pan from the heat.
4. Combine the rice with the black-bean mixture and season with salt and pepper. Divide the rice and bean mixture among 4 dinner plates. Divide the scallops into 4 portions and place on top of the rice. Garnish with parsley and serve.

■ MAKES 4 SERVINGS

The Recipes

POULTRY

ROAST CHICKEN CHEZ LOUIS

■　　■　　■

Would you like to prepare "the crustiest, juiciest, most memorable chicken this side of France" (*Town and Country* magazine); "the dewily moist, golden-skinned roast chicken . . . heady with garlic and brambly herbs" (Mimi Sheraton's *Taste*); the chicken that is "moist, with crisped skin, perfumed with garlic, and branches of rosemary and thyme" (New York *Newsday*); "herb-flecked whole chicken" that "is a delight in its simplicity" (*The New York Times*)?

This is the singular dish that put my restaurant, Chez Louis, on the culinary map of the United States and it is a natural for this program! After marinating the chicken, pat it dry; only a small amount of olive oil will adhere to the skin. The other ingredients are simply pure fresh herbs and spices and chicken stock. This dish proves that the finest cooking is also the most healthful.

MARINADE

½ cup good, full-flavored olive oil
7 cloves garlic, peeled
4 sprigs fresh thyme
4 sprigs fresh rosemary
salt and pepper to taste

One 2½- to 3-pound chicken, kosher or fresh-killed if you can get it. (There is enough marinade for two chickens if you wish to double the recipe.)
1 cup chicken stock

∎

1. Marinate the chicken(s) at least an hour in the refrigerator, and as long as overnight. Remove the chicken(s) and save the marinade. It will keep, refrigerated, up to a month.
2. Preheat the oven to its highest setting.
3. If you are going to grill the chicken in step 4, prepare a charcoal fire.
4. When the fire is ready, sear the chicken on the charcoal grill for about 3 minutes on each side. The chicken may be set aside for up to 2 hours before you proceed with the rest of the recipe. If no grill is available, you may sear the chicken in a sauté pan without any oil. You will have to double the time on each side and the flavor will not be as interesting as it will be if you sear the chicken on a grill.
5. Place the chicken in a heavy-bottomed roasting pan and roast until it is done and the juices run clear, approximately 45 minutes.
6. Remove the chicken from the roasting pan and let it rest uncovered for 10 minutes. This is done so that the meat reabsorbs its juices. Pour the excess fat from the roasting pan and deglaze the pan with chicken stock.

7 Adjust seasoning to taste.
8 Cut the chicken into serving portions. Ladle the pan juices over each serving and garnish with a sprig of watercress.

■ MAKES 4 SERVINGS

CHICKEN ROASTED ON POTATO SLICES, TOMATO SLICES, AND MASHED GARLIC

■ ■ ■

This is a great party dish, fragrant and festive, and it can be expanded easily to serve the number of people you are feeding. Your guests won't believe that there is no added fat or oil in this recipe.

2 large baking potatoes
1 fresh roasting chicken (kosher or fresh-killed if you can get it)
salt and pepper
2 large tomatoes or 8 plum tomatoes
4 cloves garlic, peeled and mashed
1 cup chicken stock
¼ cup balsamic vinegar
Tabasco sauce
2 tablespoons chopped coriander or Italian parsley

■

1. Preheat the oven to 450°F.
2. Prepare Potato Crisps according to the recipe on page 259–60. Undercook them slightly.
3. Transfer the Potato Crisps to a roasting pan large enough to hold the chicken comfortably. The potatoes can overlap.
4. Season the chicken with salt and pepper and place it on top of the layer of Potato Crisps.
5. Place the pan in the oven and roast the chicken 10 minutes on each side.
6. Add the tomatoes, garlic, chicken stock, and vinegar to the spaces around the chicken. Cover the potatoes completely.
7. Continue cooking until the chicken is done and its juices run clear, about 30 minutes. The sauce should be concentrated and somewhat lumpy.
8. Remove the chicken from the pan. Season the sauce and potato mixture to taste with salt, pepper, and Tabasco. Transfer the potato slices and sauce to a serving platter. Cut the chicken into serving pieces and place it on top of the potatoes. Sprinkle with chopped coriander or Italian parsley and serve immediately.

■ MAKES 4 SERVINGS

Roasted Chicken, Stuffed with Grilled Shiitake Mushrooms and Deglazed with Balsamic Vinegar

■ ■ ■

I often serve this knockout chicken dish at dinner parties. As I bring it to the table, its aroma is irresistible.

½ pound shiitake mushrooms, cleaned and stems removed. (Other mushrooms may be substituted.)
olive oil for brushing mushrooms
one 2½- to 3-pound chicken, kosher or fresh-killed if possible
3 tablespoons chopped shallots
½ cup balsamic vinegar
1 cup white wine
salt and pepper to taste

1. If you are going to grill the mushrooms, prepare a charcoal or wood fire. Preheat the oven to its highest possible setting.
2. Brush the mushrooms with the oil and grill them, or sear them in a hot pan, to the point that the mushroom skin has a little burn on it.
3. Season the inside of the chicken with salt and pepper. Stuff the cavity of the chicken with the grilled or seared mushrooms.
4. Place the chicken in the hot oven and turn it every 15 minutes, so that every surface browns. Cook 50 to 60 minutes.
5. Remove the chicken from the oven and place it on a platter or carving board. Tilt the roasting pan so that the fat rises to the top, and pour out the fat, reserving the juices. Place the roasting pan on the stove over medium heat and add the shallots. Stir the shallots around in the pan with a metal spatula, scraping up all the burnt particles on the bottom of the pan. Deglaze the pan with vinegar, and add the wine. Cook down the liquid, stirring and scraping with the spatula. When the sauce lightly coats a spoon, remove it from the heat and season it with salt and pepper.
6. Cut the chicken into serving portions and arrange it with the mushrooms on dinner plates. Pour the juices that have run out of the chicken into the sauce, quickly reheat the sauce, and spoon it over the top of the chicken and mushrooms.

■ MAKES 4 SERVINGS

Grilled Baby Chicken (Poussin) Stuffed with Sage

■   ■   ■

To my taste, baby chicken, also known as poussin, is much more flavorful than Cornish hen. However, either bird can become a staple in your new food repertoire. You may substitute Cornish hen in this recipe if poussin is not available.

These birds are great cooked over a fire of fruitwood. And since you have the fire going, why not make "Mickies"? For each "Mickey," wrap one potato in aluminum foil, bury it in the coals, and roast it until it is hard on the outside and soft inside.

For each serving:
1 baby chicken (poussin) about 10–12 ounces
salt and pepper to taste
1 bunch fresh sage
Tabasco sauce, optional

1. Prepare a fire of fruitwood or charcoal.
2. Season each bird with salt and pepper inside and out. Stuff the cavity with sage.
3. When the fire is ready, grill the bird. If you have the patience, use a chef's fork and turn the bird every 3 to 5 minutes from side to side, back to front, and top to bottom. This process will prevent the juices from escaping. Let the skin become a golden-brown caramelized color. When you have succeeded in browning every inch of skin, the bird is usually done. If there is a patch of raw skin, the meat will be raw underneath. This is a lot of work, but it is fun, too. The bird(s) can also be roasted in a hot oven (turned to the highest possible setting) for 25 to 30 minutes.

■ MAKES 1 SERVING

TASTY GRILLED QUAIL

Small game birds work very well on my eating plan. They are portion controlled, with one or two birds equaling one portion. It is relatively hard to get the meat off the bones, so these birds make you "sing for your supper." Serve them with quinoa, wehani rice, or Potato Crisps.

8 quail (two per person)
2 tablespoons Dijon mustard
salt and pepper to taste
3 tablespoons chopped fresh coriander or Italian parsley

1. Prepare a charcoal fire.
2. Rub the quail with salt, pepper, and mustard.
3. Grill the birds until crisp on the outside but still tender and juicy on the inside. This should take approximately 4 to 5 minutes on each side. The quail can also be broiled under a very hot broiler for about 4 minutes on each side.
4. Place the quail on a serving platter and sprinkle coriander or Italian parsley on top.

- MAKES 4 SERVINGS

TURKEY AND/OR CHICKEN BURGERS

If you decide to give up red meat, you will probably still crave an occasional thick, juicy hamburger. Turkey and chicken may be used as delicious substitutes for beef, and if you grind or chop your own, you can prepare a burger that is close to fat free.

There are endless variations to this recipe. You can add any of the following ingredients to the meat mixture:

- ½ cup onions, peppers, or mushrooms sautéed in 1 tablespoon of olive oil
- fresh mushrooms to taste
- fresh herbs to taste
- any mustard or vinegar
- minced garlic or shallots to taste

If you are on an unlimited budget, cook the burgers and then grate fresh, white truffles over the top.

Putting this dish together is like ordering a pizza—exercise your options.

1 pound ground turkey or chicken or any combination of the two. Grind the meat yourself to control the fat content.
½ cup chopped onions
3 tablespoons Dijon mustard
¼ cup balsamic vinegar
salt and pepper to taste

1. If you are going to grill the burgers, prepare a charcoal or wood fire. If you are going to broil them, preheat the broiler to very hot.
2. Combine all the ingredients and form them into 4 patties.
3. Grill, broil, or sauté the burgers in a nonstick pan. Serve plain, on warmed pita bread, or sandwiched in a crisp baked potato skin.

■ MAKES 4 SERVINGS

The Recipes

BAKED POTATO SKIN WITH GRILLED TURKEY AND ONIONS

■   ■ ■   ■

For each serving:
1 baking potato
1 tablespoon olive oil
2 slices onion
1 large slice turkey breast fillet
salt and pepper to taste
¼ cup balsamic vinegar
2 tablespoons chopped chives

■

1. Preheat the oven to its highest setting.
2. Wash and dry the potato. (Never wrap a potato in foil for baking.) Bake until the skin becomes crisp and the inside is soft. This should take about 45 minutes for a medium potato.
3. Remove the potato from the oven. Split it open and remove as much of the potato "meat" as possible. Put the skin back in the oven to keep warm.
4. Heat the oil in a nonstick pan. Add the onions and turkey to the pan and sear them on both sides. Season them with salt and

pepper, deglaze the pan with balsamic vinegar, and remove it from the heat.
5. Remove the potato skin from the oven and place it on a dish. Layer the turkey and onions inside the opened potato skin.
6. Sprinkle with the chopped chives and serve immediately.

■ MAKES 1 SERVING

The Recipes

VEGETABLES

POTATO PIE CHEZ LOUIS

This is one of the most famous recipes to come out of my New York restaurant, Chez Louis, and apparently it is talked about all over the United States. Along with Roast Chicken Chez Louis, it is the most frequently requested recipe on my menu. My inspiration for the dish came from a potato pie served at the French restaurant L'Ami Louis, but that pie is different in preparation and in end result. The recipe I give you here is for a lighter pie with a crisper exterior, and it omits one particular ingredient of the French version: goose fat. I use olive oil instead, with excellent results.

2 pounds baking potatoes
2 cloves garlic, peeled
4 tablespoons olive oil
2 tablespoons minced garlic
salt and pepper to taste
2 tablespoons chopped parsley, Italian if possible

1. Preheat the oven to its highest setting.
2. In a large pot, boil the potatoes in salted water with the 2 cloves of garlic until potatoes are tender, about 20 to 25 minutes.
3. Drain the potatoes and set them aside until they are cool enough to handle. Cut them into ¼-inch slices. Do not peel them. Discard the garlic.
4. Heat the olive oil with the minced garlic in a sauté pan and sauté the potato slices until they are lightly browned. Season them with salt and pepper while they cook.
5. Arrange the potato slices in a very clean, lightly oiled, 9-inch black cast-iron skillet. Press the slices down firmly with the back of a spoon or with a clean dish towel. They should hold together in a "pie."
6. Place the potatoes in the oven and bake for 20 to 25 minutes until they are crispy on the outside. You may wish to bake them a few minutes longer for an especially crisp exterior. A very crisp potato pie will be brown in color.
7. Remove the skillet from the oven. Slide a spatula under the pie and invert it onto a serving plate. Garnish with parsley. Serve immediately.

■ MAKES 4–6 SERVINGS

POTATO PIE WITH CLAMS AND CORIANDER

∎   ∎   ∎

2 pounds baking potatoes
2 cloves garlic, peeled
2 tablespoons minced garlic
4 tablespoons olive oil
salt and pepper to taste
2 tablespoons minced shallots
½ pound fresh, frozen, or canned clams
2 tablespoons chopped coriander

∎

1. Preheat the oven to its highest setting.
2. In a large pot, boil the potatoes and garlic cloves in salted water until the potatoes are tender, about 20 to 25 minutes.
3. Drain the potatoes and set them aside until they are cool enough to handle. Cut them into ¼-inch slices. Do not peel them. Discard the garlic.
4. Heat the oil in a sauté pan and add the minced garlic. Sauté the potato slices until they are lightly browned. Season the potatoes with salt and pepper to taste while they cook.
5. Arrange ½ of the potato slices in a very clean, lightly oiled, 9-inch black cast-iron skillet. Mix together the shallots and clams in a small bowl. Spoon the clam mixture evenly over the potato

slices. Arrange the remaining potato slices on top of the clams. Press the slices down firmly with the back of a spoon or with a clean dish towel. They should hold together in a "pie."
6. Place the potatoes in the oven and bake for 20 to 25 minutes until they are crispy on the outside. You may wish to bake them a few minutes longer for an especially crisp exterior. A very crisp potato pie will be brown in color.
7. Remove the skillet from the oven. Slide a spatula under the pie and invert it onto a serving plate. Garnish with parsley and serve immediately.

◾ MAKES 4–6 SERVINGS

The Recipes

ROASTED MUSHROOMS AND GARLIC CHEZ LOUIS

Exotic mushrooms are ideal in this recipe, although domestic mushrooms also make a delicious version. Shiitakes and pleurottes are becoming available in many markets all year long. In fact, the Campbell Soup Company is cultivating such mushrooms and selling them in supermarkets under the names "Imperials" and "Oysters." The even more exotic cepes and chanterelles appear in many shops in the fall.

6–8 cloves garlic, unpeeled
1 pound mushrooms, stems removed
4 branches fresh thyme or ½ teaspoon dry thyme leaves
3 tablespoons mild olive oil mixed with 4 cloves garlic, peeled and mashed
2 tablespoons red wine vinegar
salt and pepper to taste

1   Heat the oven to 350°F and roast the garlic cloves for 30 minutes.

2. Place the roasted garlic cloves and the mushrooms in an even layer in a heavy baking dish. Place the thyme on top of the garlic and mushrooms.
3. Brush the oil and raw garlic mixture on the mushrooms and garlic cloves. Sprinkle the red wine vinegar over all. Season with salt and pepper to taste.
4. Place in the 350°F oven and bake 20 minutes.
5. Serve with good French bread to sop up the juices. The soft interior of the roasted garlic cloves may be spread on the bread or eaten with the mushrooms.

■ MAKES 4 SERVINGS

The Recipes

ROASTED VEGETABLES

■   ■   ■

This vegetable combination has been a standby of my program and can be served as a main dish or a side dish. You can include any fresh vegetables that look good and you can vary the ingredients with the seasons. There are no rules about what goes with what. The only rule is: The fresher the vegetables, the better the dish.

4 medium onions, peeled and quartered
8 medium carrots, scraped
4 medium turnips, scraped and quartered
4 medium beets, peeled and quartered
1 head garlic, broken up but with individual cloves left unpeeled
4 small zucchini or yellow squash cut in half lengthwise
any other fresh vegetables that look interesting
2 tablespoons olive oil
salt and pepper to taste

■

1   Preheat the oven to its highest setting.
2   Rub all the vegetables with a small amount of oil—a little goes a long way. Season the vegetables with salt and pepper.

3. Place the vegetables in a heavy-bottomed roasting pan. Turn them frequently while they are roasting so that they brown evenly on all sides and get nice and crusty. Roast for about 35 minutes. The garlic "meat" is delicious spread on a crust of bread.

■ MAKES 4 SERVINGS

BAKED POTATO WITH SALSA AND SEARED SHRIMP

The versatile baked potato is a staple of this food program. It can serve as a fallback food, as a simple lunch, or as a little "dinner before you eat dinner." Here it is topped with shrimp and a spicy, low-calorie, fat-free salsa.

For each portion:
1 baking potato, washed well
½ cup chopped fresh tomato
2 tablespoons chopped green chili peppers (add more if you want the salsa to be hotter)
1 cup minced onions
3 tablespoons minced shallots
1 tablespoon lemon juice
salt and pepper to taste
¼ pound shrimp, shelled and deveined

■

1. Preheat the oven to its highest setting.
2. Bake the potato until the skin is crisp and the inside is soft, about 45 minutes for a medium potato. Never wrap a potato in foil for baking.
3. Combine all the other ingredients except the shrimp in a stainless steel, china, or glass bowl to make the salsa.
4. Heat a nonstick sauté pan and sear the shrimp for 2 minutes on each side. Remove the shrimp from the heat.
5. Remove the potato from the oven, break it open, and spoon the salsa on top. Arrange the shrimp over the salsa.

■ MAKES 1 SERVING

KILLER POTATOES WITH HOT CHILIES

■   ■   ■

The key to this recipe is to cook the potatoes over low heat for a long period of time, so that they get very crisp on the outside while they stay moist inside. You may increase the amount of chili peppers if you like your food especially hot.

4 medium baking potatoes
4 tablespoons good-quality olive oil
4 tablespoons minced hot chili peppers
4 tablespoons chopped shallots
salt and pepper to taste

■

1. Wash and dry the potatoes, but do not peel them. Cut them into 1-inch chunks. Cover the potatoes with a dry cloth while you prepare the chilies.
2. Heat the olive oil in a large nonstick sauté pan. Sauté the chilies and the shallots together for 4 to 7 minutes. Make sure the heat is medium low.

The Recipes

3. Add the potatoes to the pan. Cook them, tossing and turning them so that all sides are exposed to the hot oil. The potatoes should be cooked in 45 minutes to 1 hour. They should be brown and crisp.
4. Transfer the potatoes to a serving bowl. Scrape the chilies and shallots from the bottom of the pan over the potatoes. Season with salt and pepper and serve.

■ MAKES 4 SERVINGS

CHINESE GARLIC BROCCOLI

■   ■   ■

1 bunch broccoli
6 cloves garlic, peeled
1 cup chicken stock
salt and pepper to taste

■

1. Wash the broccoli and cut it into manageable pieces.
2. Mash the garlic. Combine the garlic and the chicken stock in a sauté pan and bring to a boil.

3. Lower the heat and add the broccoli to the stock. Cover the pan and simmer 7 minutes or until the broccoli is tender.
4. Remove the broccoli to a serving platter. Reduce the liquid by half and pour it over the broccoli. Season with salt and pepper. Sprinkle the garlic over the top.

■ MAKES 4 SERVINGS

STEAMED CABBAGE WITH CHINESE BLACK BEANS

This a great vegetable dish that is easy to make. Because of its spicy flavor and chunky texture, it goes beautifully with plain roasted chicken. Chinese cabbage (bok choy) is more flavorful than regular cabbage and doesn't get rubbery when it is steamed.

1 small head Chinese cabbage, approximately 2 pounds
2 tablespoons olive oil
3 tablespoons chopped shallots

½ cup Chinese black beans (available in Asian markets and some supermarkets)
1 teaspoon Chinese chili paste or to taste (it is quite spicy)
1 cup chicken stock
salt and pepper to taste

■

1. Wash the cabbage well and slice it into ½-inch strips.
2. Heat the olive oil in a sauté pan and sauté the shallots 5 to 7 minutes. Add the black beans. Pour the shallots, beans, and cabbage into a large pot and mix well. Add the chicken stock, and bring it to a boil. Add the chili paste. Steam the vegetables until the cabbage is tender, about 10 minutes.
3. Transfer the cabbage to a serving bowl. Pour the black bean mixture on top. Season with salt and pepper and serve.

■ MAKES 4 SERVINGS

Crusty Brown Rice with Vegetables

■   ■   ■

This dish, a healthful, low-fat version of Chinese fried rice, can be prepared days in advance and cooked when needed. Simply complete the recipe up to step 4 and refrigerate the rice mixture until you are ready to cook it. If you like food hot and spicy, substitute hot pepper oil for the olive oil.

This is a perfect example of a mix-and-match recipe. You can add any vegetables you like, or even substitute different kinds of rice.

1 cup brown rice or wehani rice
2 tablespoons olive oil or 2 tablespoons Chinese hot pepper oil
½ cup diced onions
2 tablespoons minced shallots
½ cup diced celery
½ cup diced carrots
½ cup diced radishes
salt and pepper to taste

1. Bring 2 cups water to a boil, add the brown rice, cover, and simmer over low heat for 35 to 40 minutes, or until the rice has absorbed all the water.
2. Heat the oil in a nonstick sauté pan, add the onion and shallot, and cook for 5 minutes over low heat. Add the rest of the vegetables and cook, stirring, for an additional 10 minutes, until lightly browned.
3. Transfer the rice to the sauté pan, mix it well with the vegetables, and season the mixture with salt and pepper.
4. Using a spatula, press down hard on the rice, forcing it into a pancake shape.
5. Lower the heat and cook the rice and vegetable mixture until the bottom is crisp, about 15 minutes. Turn and cook it until the other side is crisp, another 15 minutes.
6. Slide the "crusty" rice out of the pan and onto a serving plate. The concoction should look like Egg Foo Yung without sauce.

■ MAKES 4 SERVINGS

LENTILS WITH VEGETABLES

■   ■   ■

This dish requires a long cooking time but it is a great fallback food to keep in your refrigerator. I recommend Legumor French green lentils, which I think are the best even though preparing them requires patience. If you can't find this brand, substitute another. You will find the cooking times differ for other brands; check the directions on the package.

10 ounces lentils
2 tablespoons olive oil
½ cup minced onions
2 tablespoons minced shallots
½ cup minced carrots
salt and pepper to taste
Tabasco sauce, optional
2 tablespoons chopped coriander or Italian parsley

■

1   Bring a large pot of water to a boil. Wash the lentils and add them to the pot. Cover and simmer for 1½ hours or as directed on the package.

2. When the lentils are done, drain them and set aside.
3. Heat the olive oil in a sauté pan and sauté the onions, shallots, and carrots for 10 minutes over medium heat.
4. Add the lentils to the pan. Combine everything well and season with salt and pepper. Add Tabasco if you like a spicier flavor. Sprinkle with chopped coriander or Italian parsley.

■ MAKES 4 SERVINGS

CONDIMENTS

TAPENADE

This is a good-stuff mixture: it contains capers, olives, garlic, and anchovies. I like the flavors of the individual ingredients and the flavor that results when the ingredients are combined. And it has the rough, interesting texture of a peasant dish.

Tapenade has endless simple uses. It is delicious spread on a crust of French or Italian bread. I rub it into the skin of a chicken either before or after grilling and I use it to coat a piece of fish that I then grill or sauté. I also spread it on fish after cooking. I mix it into a pasta dish or use it as the sole flavoring for pasta. It is interesting cooked, because it gets crusty on the grilled chicken or fish, and equally interesting uncooked.

This is a flexible recipe that you can adjust to your own taste. If you want to tone down the anchovy flavor, simply decrease the amount. Add or subtract garlic and spices, if you like. Use tapenade sparingly— a little goes a long way. It can be stored in the refrigerator, tightly covered, for months.

¼ cup pitted Niçoise olives
6 anchovies, chopped
2 tablespoons olive oil
2 tablespoons capers
2 cloves garlic, peeled and mashed
1 tablespoon lemon juice
salt and pepper to taste
cayenne pepper or hot pepper sauce to taste

1. Place all the ingredients except the spices in a food processor and process until the mixture has the consistency of a rough paste. Remove the tapenade and season it.
2. Store the tapenade in a sealable container in the refrigerator until you are ready to use it.

MAKES ½ CUP

Apple Cider Jelly

Make this jelly and store it in the refrigerator—it will be the basis of many interesting light desserts. It can last almost indefinitely in a tightly closed container. If a little mold begins to form on the top surface, simply scrape it away—the jelly underneath will be fine. Apple cider jelly can be used as a sweetener in just about anything, and it contains no sugar other than the sucrose occurring naturally in the apple cider.

1 gallon unfiltered fresh apple cider, with no preservatives added

1. Bring the cider to a boil in a large pot. Lower the heat and simmer the cider until it is reduced to 2 pints (32 ounces). That is, reduce it 8 to 1.
2. Let the cider cool at room temperature.
3. Store in a sealed container and refrigerate.

■ MAKES 2 PINTS

The Recipes

FRUIT

Apples Baked with Apple Cider Jelly and Cinnamon

■   ■   ■

If you must eat a dessert, this one is about as guilt free as they come. It is equally good eaten hot or cold.

4 medium apples—Macintosh and Mutsus are good
1 cup apple cider jelly
1 tablespoon cinnamon

■

1. Preheat the oven to 375°F.
2. Core each apple.
3. Combine the apple cider jelly and the cinnamon.

4   Place the apples on a nonstick baking pan. Spoon the jelly mixture into the core of each apple and bake the apples for 30 minutes. Bake longer if you like the apples very soft.

■ MAKES 4 SERVINGS

FRUIT FLOATING IN FRUIT

This looks and tastes like a "real" dessert, but it is as close to fresh fruit as you can get. If the fruit is not absolutely ripe, the combination will not work.

4 large ripe peaches (white are the best)
¼ cup apple cider jelly
1 tablespoon pure vanilla extract
2 pints strawberries
mint sprigs for garnish

1. Core the peaches but do not peel them. Purée them, with the jelly and vanilla extract, in a food processor.
2. Wash and stem the strawberries and cut each berry in half.
3. Pour ¼ of the peach purée in each of four dessert bowls. Top with ¼ of the strawberries. Garnish each bowl with a mint sprig.

■ MAKES 4 SERVINGS

NO-CHOLESTEROL STRAWBERRY TART/PIE

I am not saying that this tart/pie has no calories! But it is cholesterol free and it contains no sugar other than the fructose occurring naturally in the strawberries and apple cider jelly. It is a beautiful dessert to serve at a dinner party—I guarantee that it will be a conversation piece.

1⅓ cups unsifted all-purpose flour
12 tablespoons chilled tub margarine
2 teaspoons salt
3 tablespoons ice water
4 pounds very ripe strawberries
½ cup apple cider jelly

■

1. Preheat the oven to 300°F.
2. Combine the flour, margarine, and salt in a food processor. Process until the mixture resembles oatmeal. Drizzle the ice water through the top opening while the machine is running, until a doughball forms and the exterior looks smooth. Wrap the doughball in waxed paper and refrigerate it for 2 hours. This dough can be made and refrigerated up to 7 days in advance.
3. While the dough is resting, wash and stem the strawberries. Chop 1 pound of the strawberries into a rough paste and combine with the apple cider jelly. Reserve the remaining berries.
4. After the dough has rested, roll it out ⅛ inch to ¼ inch thick and transfer it to a pie pan. Crimp the edges with your fingers to give the crust a professional look. If you prefer to make a tart, roll the dough into a rectangle approximately 10 inches by 10 inches, or into any shape you choose, as long as it remains ⅛ inch to ¼ inch thick. Place it on a nonstick baking surface and crimp the edges.
5. Bake the crust for 30 minutes. Remove it from the oven, spread the strawberry and jelly mixture over it, and bake it for another 30 minutes, or until the crust is nut brown all the way through. (This is low-heat baking.) Remove it from the oven.
6. Arrange the remaining 2 pounds of whole strawberries on top of the pie/tart in a tightly packed pattern. Either serve the

dessert immediately or prepare it in advance and serve it after dinner.

- MAKES 1 10-INCH ROUND PIE OR 1 TART APPROXIMATELY 10 INCHES BY 10 INCHES. SIZES ARE NOT EXACT.

SNACKS AND FALLBACKS

SPICY POPCORN

Freezing popcorn before popping it gives you a much fluffier product. When the cold popcorn hits the very hot pan, pressure builds up internally and the outer kernel explodes with extra power. For that spicy flavor, I like to use Konriko Cajun spice, a brand that is available in many stores and that contains no MSG.

1 cup popcorn
1 tablespoon olive oil
black pepper to taste
Cajun spice (Konriko) to taste, or cayenne pepper or onion powder to taste

1. Freeze popcorn for a half hour.
2. Combine the oil, pepper, and spice in a heavy pot or corn popper.

3 Add the frozen popcorn and stir well.
4 If you are using a pot, cook the popcorn, covered, over low heat 8 to 10 minutes or until it has all popped. If you are using a corn popper, follow the manufacturer's directions.

Note: When you use a heavy pot to pop the corn, keep the heat low and the popping process slow. The longer the popping time, the fluffier the popcorn.

■ MAKES ABOUT 1 GALLON

POTATO CRISPS

■ ■ ■

Potato crisps are my personal miracle food. Since I began this program, I have relied on this dish whenever I have felt the need for something crunchy and tasty to eat on relatively short notice. I would rather snack on potato crisps than almost anything I can think of.

Potato crisps also make an excellent side dish for the chicken and fish recipes you will find in this book. They can be made in advance and reheated, or they can be sliced in advance, covered well to keep out the air, and baked at the last minute.

1 large baking potato
salt, pepper, or Cajun spice to taste

■

1. Heat the oven to 450°F.
2. Wash and dry the potato well; do not peel it.
3. Slice the potato into ⅛-inch pieces.
4. You will need a large nonstick baking sheet or a regular baking sheet lined with parchment paper. Arrange the slices on a baking sheet so that they do not overlap. Season them to taste.
5. Bake 7 minutes or until the potato slices are browned and crisp. Turn and bake another 7 minutes.
6. Remove the potato crisps from the oven and serve immediately.

■ YIELD DEPENDS UPON HOW THIN YOU SLICE THE POTATO.

The Recipes

MUFFINS AND COOKIES

DAVID'S OAT-BRAN MUFFINS

■   ■   ■

These are the famous muffins that were named most nutritious ounce for ounce by *The New York Times* in November 1988. What makes them different from any other oat-bran muffins on the market, as far as I know, is that they are the only tasty muffins available that have absolutely no fat added. The minute quantity of fat in the muffin occurs naturally in the oat bran itself.

It is important to remember two things when you prepare these muffins: use foil muffin cups so the oil-free mixture will not stick to the cups; and bake the muffins immediately upon mixing the ingredients, or else the batter will turn to sludge before your eyes.

If oat bran isn't available, you can substitute dry oatmeal. And be sure to try some of my delicious variations on the original muffin.

2 cups oat bran (or dry oatmeal)
⅓ cup unbleached all-purpose flour
¼ teaspoon baking powder
½ teaspoon baking soda
½ teaspoon salt
½ teaspoon cinnamon
¼ teaspoon allspice
10 ounces skim milk
Egg whites from 2 large eggs
5 ounces apple cider jelly or sugar-free fruit preserves, such as Smucker's, Sorrel Ridge, or Polaner'. The fruit preserves come in 10-ounce jars; use ½ jar.
¾ cup raisins

1. Preheat the oven to 350°F.
2. Combine all the dry ingredients.
3. Mix in all the remaining ingredients. This is a very wet batter, and you need not worry about overmixing it.
4. Spoon the batter into 2½-ounce foil muffin cups set into muffin pans. Bake 22 minutes or until the muffins are brown and firm.

Variations: For a chunkier—and sometimes higher calorie—muffin, add 1 cup dried fruit chunks to the batter. Use dried pineapple, apricots, or any fruit desired.

■ MAKES 14–18 MUFFINS

The Recipes

DAVID'S OAT-BRAN COOKIES

■   ■   ■

If you want a change from oat-bran muffins, you can get your daily allotment of oat bran in a chewy, delicious cookie. Four cookies each day will provide the recommended amount. These treats look something like peanut-butter cookies and taste like oatmeal-spice cookies.

2¾ cups oat bran
10 ounces (1 jar) sugar-free fruit preserves (Smucker's, Sorrel Ridge, or Polaner')
4 ounces safflower oil
1 cup unbleached all-purpose flour
Egg whites from 3 large eggs
1 cup raisins
2 teaspoons cinnamon
2 teaspoons vanilla extract
½ teaspoon baking soda
1 teaspoon salt

■

1. Preheat the oven to 325°F.
2. Drop the batter by tablespoonfuls onto a nonstick baking sheet or a regular baking sheet spread with parchment. Press the cookies down with a moistened fork to even them out. The batter will be wet and sloppy.
3. Bake the cookies for 9 to 10 minutes or until set.

■ MAKES 24 3-INCH COOKIES

INDEX

Aerobic exercise, 107–8
Aerobics (Cooper), 108
Aerobics Program for Total Well-Being, The (Cooper), 108
Air Force Diet, 36
Airline food, 153–54
Alcohol, 55–56
All or nothing concept, 40
Anchovies
  Linguine with Garlic and, 200–1
  Tapenade, 250–51
Anderson, Dr. James, 66
Apple
  Baked, 253
  Cider Jelly, 252
Arthur Bryant's, 23
Atkins, Dr. Robert C., 36

Baked
  Apples, 253
  Potato Skin with Grilled Turkey and Onions, 70, 231–32
Black Bean(s)
  with Grilled or Seared Shrimp, 214–15
  Soup, 181–82
  Steamed Cabbage with Chinese, 244–45
  Whole-Wheat Pasta Elbows with Shrimp, Crab, Peas and, 196–97
Black Olive
  and Mushroom Pizza, 208
Bread, 88
Breakfast, 90–91, 96
Bridge foods, 8, 40, 93, 125
Broccoli
  Chinese Garlic, 243–44
  Steamed, with Grilled Shrimp, 213–14
Brown rice, 88
  Crusty, with Vegetables, 246–47
Burgers
  Chicken or Turkey, 229–30

Cabbage
  Steamed, with Chinese Black Beans, 244–45
Calisthenics, 108
Calorie(s)
  counting, 37–38
  and food decisions, 69–70
  in oils, 65
Canola oil, 65
Capers, 250

Index

Chicken
 Burgers, 229–30
 Grilled Baby (Poussin), Stuffed with Sage, 227–28
 Roasted
  Chez Louis, 221–22
  on Potato Slices, Tomato Slices, and Mashed Garlic, 223–24
  Salad, 189–90
  Stuffed with Grilled Shiitake Mushrooms and Deglazed with Balsamic Vinegar, 225–26
 stock and reduction, 173–79
Chilies, Killer Potatoes with Hot, 242–43
Chinese
 Garlic Broccoli, 243–44
 restaurants, 139
Cholesterol, 60–73, 75, 76
 and exercise, 104, 107
 HDL vs. LDL, 64, 65, 66, 104
 modification, 6, 7–8
Cholesterol: Your Guide For A Healthy Heart, 64
Chunky Tuna Salad, 190–91
Clam
 Potato Pie with Coriander and, 235–36
 White, Pizza, 206–7
Clothing, 28–29
Coffee shops and diners, 141–42
Compulsive eating, 10–31
 breaking compulsion, 29–30
 controlling, 6–7
 defined, 4–6
 monitoring, 8
Cookies
 Oat Bran, 263–64
Cooking, 159–73

Cooking the Nouvelle Cuisine in America (Liederman and Urvater), 19, 159
Cooper, Dr. Kenneth H., 107, 108
Cornish Hen Stuffed with Sage, 227–28
Corn oil, 65
Crab
 Whole-Wheat Pasta Elbows with Shrimp, Black Beans, Peas and, 196–97
Crusty Brown Rice with Vegetables, 246–47

David's
 Breakfast, 91
 French Bread Pizza Dough, 203–5
 Oat-Bran Muffins, 261–62
 Endless-Variation Pasta, 193–95
Deglazing, 168
Delicatessens, 142
Delicious weight-loss program, 8, 30, 74–101
Diets, 7, 35–43, 74–75
Dinner, 92, 96, 97, 98, 99
 "eating," before dinner, 126–27, 134
Drinking Man's Diet, 35–36

8-Week Cholesterol Cure, The (Kowalski), 64
Endive and Watercress Salad with Walnuts and Parmesan, 186–87
Equipment, 166
Excuses, 130–31
Exercise, 8, 30, 42, 100, 102–15
 and cholesterol, 73
 compulsive, 114–15

Fast food, 142

Index

Fats, 65–66, 161
Feeding others, 122–24
Fiber, 66, 87–89
  insoluble, 66, 69
  soluble, 66, 69
  sources, 88–89
Fine cooking, 6, 7
Fish stock and reduction, 174–76
Food
  buddy, 128–29
  decisions, and variables, 69–73
  fallbacks, 8, 125–26
  journal, 8, 30, 41, 100, 117–21
Ford, Charlotte, 150
French Bread Pizza Dough, 203–5
French restaurants, 137
Fruit Floating in Fruit, 254–55

Garlic
  Broccoli, Chinese, 243–44
  Linguine with Anchovies and, 200–1
  Roasted Chicken, on Potato Slices, Tomato Slices, and, 223–24
  Roasted Mushrooms and, 237–38
Goldberg, Larry "Fats," 23–24
Golden Rules, 100–1
Grapefruit Diet, 36
Green Peas "French style," 71
Grilling, 167
Guide Michelin, 19

Hazen, Marcella, 138
Hearty Turkey and Potato Soup, 184–85
Hot Fudge Sunday Diet, 36
Hydrogenated oil, 65, 69

Ice cream, 54–55
  ersatz, 54–55

Indian restaurants, 140
Italian restaurants, 138

Japanese restaurants, 139
Jelly, Apple Cider, 252

Kansas City, 23–24
Killer Potatoes with Hot Chilies, 242–43
Kitchen
  cleaning out, 81

Leeks
  Melted, on Swordfish, 210–11
  Pasta with Grilled Shrimp, Shiitake Mushrooms and, 200–1
Lentils with Vegetables, 248–49
Life change, 41
Linguine with Garlic and Anchovies, 201–2
Lobster
  Roasted with Tarragon, 217–18
  Salad, 187–88
Lunch, 91–92, 97, 98

Marinade
  for Roast Chicken, 222
Marinating, 169
Menus, 95–100
Methods, 167–69
Mexican restaurants, 140
Monounsaturated fats, 65, 69
Muffins
  David's Oat-Bran, 261—62
Mushroom
  with Grilled Shrimp, Leeks, and Pasta, 200–1
  Pizza with Black Olives and, 208
  Roasted
    Chicken Stuffed with, 225–26

Index

Mushroom (cont.)
    with Garlic, 237–38
    and Scallops on Spicy Rice, 219–20
    Soup, 184–85
Mussels, Shallots, and Coriander in Spicy Broth, 216–17
Mustard Vinaigrette, 187

New Aerobics, The (Cooper), 107
No list, 77–78, 83, 89–90
No-Oil Vinaigrette, 192

Oat bran, 7, 8, 66–67, 87–88
    Cookies, 263–64
    Muffins, 67–68, 261–62
Olive oil, 65
Onions
    Baked Potato Skin with Grilled Turkey and, 231–32
    Tuna Seared with Mustard and, 212–13
    Whole-Wheat Pasta with Tomatoes, Capers, and, 198–99

Parties, 8
    eating wisely at, 149–51
Pasta, 164–65
    Endless-Variation, 193–95
    with Grilled Shrimp, Leeks, and Shiitake Mushrooms, 200–1
    Linguine with Garlic and Anchovies, 201–2
    Whole-Wheat
        Elbows with Shrimp, Crab, Black Beans and Peas, 196–97
        with Tomatoes, Capers, and Onions, 198–99
Peaches, 254–55
Peanut oil, 65

Peas
    Whole-Wheat Pasta Elbows with Shrimp, Crab, Black Beans and, 196–97
Pepe's pizza, 24
Pie
    Potato
        Chez Louis, 233–34
        with Clams and Coriander, 235–36
    Strawberry No-Cholesterol, 255–56
Pizza
    Cheeseless Wild Mushroom and Black Olive, 208
    dough, 203–5
    White-Clam, 206–7
Plateaus, 94–95
Point, Fernand, 27
Polyunsaturated fats, 65, 69
Popcorn
    Diet, 37
    Spicy, 258–59
Positive habits, 127
Potato(es)
    Baked
        with Salsa and Seared Shrimp, 240–41
        Skin with Grilled Turkey and Onions, 231–32
    Chicken Roasted on, with Tomato and Garlic, 223–24
    Crisps, 259–60
    Hot Chilies with, 242–43
    Pie
        Chez Louis, 233–34
        with Clams and Coriander, 235–36
    Soup, with Turkey, 184–85
Poussin Stuffed with Sage, 227–28

Quail, Grilled, 228–29
Quinoa, 88, 164

Index

Recipes, 9
Red meat, 76
Reducing a sauce, 168–69
Refusing harmful foods, 124–25
Restaurant Chapel, 20
Restaurant Pic, 22
Restaurant Pyramide, 20
Restaurant Troisgros, 18–19, 132
Restaurants, 8
  eating in, wisely, 132–49
  three-star, 19–20, 147–48
Rice, 88
  Crusty, with Vegetables, 246–47
  Mussels, Shallots, and Coriander in Spicy Broth with, 216–17
  Spicy, Crispy Scallops and Mushrooms on, 219–20
Roast
  Chicken
    Chez Louis, 221–22
    on Potato Slices, Tomato Slices, and Mashed Garlic, 223–24
    Salad, 189–90
    Stuffed with Shiitake Mushrooms and Deglazed with Balsamic Vinegar, 225–26
  Mushrooms and Garlic, 237–38
  Vegetables, 239–40
Roasting, 168

Safflower oil, 65
Salad
  Chunky Tuna, 190–91
  Lobster or Shrimp, 187–88
  Roasted Chicken, 189–90
  Watercress and Endive, 186–87
Salad Dressing
  Mustard Vinaigrette, 187
  No-Oil Vinaigrette, 192

Salsa
  Baked Potato with Seared Shrimp and, 240–41
Salt, 161
Satiation, 40
Sauces
  building, 169
  reducing, 168
Sautéing, 167
Saturated fats, 64–65, 69, 76, 89
Scallops
  Baked in Shells, 72
  Crispy, with Mushrooms on Spicy Rice, 219–20
Searing, 167
Sesame oil, 65
Shrimp
  Grilled or Seared
    with Baked Potato and Salsa, 240–41
    with Black Bean Sauce, 214–15
    with Pasta, Leeks, and Shiitake Mushrooms, 200–1
    with Steamed Broccoli, 213–14
  Salad, 187–88
  Whole-Wheat Pasta Elbows with Crab, Black Beans, Peas and, 196–97
Slow Richard's, 24
Snacks, 93
Soup
  Black Bean, 181–82
  Chicken stock, 176–79
  Fish stock, 174–76
  Mussels, Shallots, and Coriander in Spicy Broth, 216–17
  Turkey and Potato, 184–85
  White Bean, 180–81
  Wild Mushroom, 183–84
Soybean oil, 65
Spas, 113–14

Index

Spicy Popcorn, 258–59
Sports food, 151–53
Staples, 165
Steamed Cabbage with Chinese Black Beans, 244–45
Stocks and reductions, 173–79
Strategies to stay on track, 124–31
Strawberries
  Fruit Floating with Fruit, 254
  No-Cholesterol Tart/Pie, 255–57
Stroud's, 24
Sunflower oil, 65
Sweating, 167
Swordfish
  Grilled or Broiled on Melted Leeks, 210–11
  Spicy, Grilled or Seared, 209–10

Tapenade, 250–51
Tart
  No-Cholesterol Strawberry, 255–57
Thai restaurants, 140–41
Tomatoes
  Chicken Roasted on, with Potato Slices and Garlic, 223–24
  Whole-Wheat Pasta with Capers, Onions, and, 198–99
Traveling, 8
  and exercise, 112–13
Trigger foods, 7, 30, 40, 47–59, 68, 69, 76–77, 83, 89, 100
  eliminating, 50–53
Trigger situations, 56–58
Trillin, Calvin, 23
Tuna
  Chunky Salad, 190–91
  Seared with Mustard and Onions, 212–13

Turkey
  or Chicken Burgers, 229–30
  Grilled, with Baked Potato Skin and Onions, 231–32
  and Potato Soup, 184–85

Urvater, Michèle, 19, 159

Veal, 89
Vegetables,
  with Crusty Brown Rice, 246–47
  Lentils with, 248–49
  Roasted, 239–40
Video tapes, exercise, 111–12
Vietnamese restaurants, 140–41
Vinaigrette
  Mustard, 187
  No-Oil, 192

Walnut oil, 65
Watercress and Endive Salad with Walnuts and Parmesan, 186–87
Wehani rice, 88, 164
Weight Watchers' Diet, 37
White Bean Soup, 180–81
White-Clam Pizza, 206–7
Whole-Wheat Pasta
  Elbows with Shrimp, Crab, Black Beans and Peas, 196–97
  with Tomatoes, Capers, and Onions, 198–99
Wild Mushroom
  Pizza, with Black Olives, 208
  Soup, 183–84
Winkler, Stacy and Henry, 149
Women
  and compulsive eating, 41–43

Yes list, 82, 87–89

COOKING? DIETING? HERE'S HELP!

THE FOOD ALLERGY COOKBOOK
Allergy Information Association
_____ 90185-2 $4.95 U.S.

EASY, SWEET AND SUGARFREE
Karne E. Barkie
_____ 90282-4 $3.50 U.S.   _____ 90283-2 $4.50 Can.

BLOOMINGDALE'S EAT HEALTHY DIET
Laura Stein
_____ 90641-2 $3.95 U.S.   _____ 90642-0 $4.95 Can.

MARY ELLEN'S HELP YOURSELF DIET PLAN
Mary Ellen Pinkham
_____ 90237-9 $2.95 U.S.   _____ 90238-7 $3.95 Can.

THE BOOK OF WHOLE GRAINS
Marlene Anne Bumgarner
_____ 92411-9 $4.95 U.S.   _____ $5.95 Can.

Publishers Book and Audio Mailing Service
P.O. Box 120159, Staten Island, NY 10312-0004

Please send me the book(s) I have checked above. I am enclosing $_____
(please add $1.25 for the first book, and $.25 for each additional book to cover postage and handling. Send check or money order only—no CODs) or charge my VISA, MASTERCARD or AMERICAN EXPRESS card.

Card number _____

Expiration date _____ Signature _____

Name _____
Address _____
City _____ State/Zip _____

Please allow six weeks for delivery. Prices subject to change without notice. Payment in U.S. funds only. New York residents add applicable sales tax.

CD 10/89

HERE'S HOW

HOW TO BUY A CAR by James R. Ross
The essential guide that gives you the edge in buying a new or used car.
_____ 90198-4 $3.95 U.S.   _____ 90199-2 $4.95 Can.

THE WHOLESALE-BY-MAIL CATALOG—UPDATE 1986 by The Print Project
Everything you need at 30% to 90% off retail prices—by mail or phone!
_____ 90379-0 $3.95 U.S.   _____ 90380-4 $4.95 Can.

TAKING CARE OF CLOTHES: An Owner's Manual for Care, Repair and Spot Removal by Mablen Jones
The most comprehensive handbook of its kind...save money—and save your wardrobe!
_____ 90355-3 $4.95 U.S.   _____ 90356-1 $5.95 Can.

AND THE LUCKY WINNER IS...The Complete Guide to Winning Sweepstakes & Contests
by Carolyn and Roger Tyndall with Tad Tyndall
Increase the odds in your favor—all you need to know.
_____ 90025-2 $3.95 U.S.   _____ 90026-0 $4.95 Can.

THE OFFICIAL HARVARD STUDENT AGENCIES BARTENDING COURSE
The new complete guide to drinkmaking—the $40 course now a paperback book!
_____ 90427-4 $3.95 U.S.   _____ 90430-4 $4.95 Can.

Publishers Book and Audio Mailing Service
P.O. Box 120159, Staten Island, NY 10312-0004

Please send me the book(s) I have checked above. I am enclosing $_____ (please add $1.25 for the first book, and $.25 for each additional book to cover postage and handling. Send check or money order only—no CODs) or charge my VISA, MASTERCARD or AMERICAN EXPRESS card.

Card number _____

Expiration date _____ Signature _____

Name _____

Address _____

City _____ State/Zip _____

Please allow six weeks for delivery. Prices subject to change without notice. Payment in U.S. funds only. New York residents add applicable sales tax.

TACKLE LIFE'S PROBLEMS

With Help From St. Martin's Paperbacks!

HOW TO LOVE A DIFFICULT MAN
Nancy Good
_____ 90963-2 $3.95 U.S. _____ 90964-0 $4.95 Can.

BEYOND CINDERELLA
Nita Tucker with Debra Feinstein
_____ 91161-0 $3.95 U.S. _____ 91162-9 $4.95 Can.

WHEN YOUR CHILD DRIVES YOU CRAZY
Eda Le Shan
_____ 90387-1 $4.95 U.S. _____ 90392-8 $5.95 Can.

HOW TO GET A MAN TO MAKE A COMMITMENT
Bonnie Barnes & Tisha Clark
_____ 90189-5 $3.95 U.S. _____ 90190-9 $4.95 Can.

HAVE A LOVE AFFAIR WITH YOUR HUSBAND
Susan Kohl & Alice Bregman
_____ 91037-1 $3.50 U.S. _____ 91039-8 $4.50 Can.

Publishers Book and Audio Mailing Service
P.O. Box 120159, Staten Island, NY 10312-0004

Please send me the book(s) I have checked above. I am enclosing $_____ (please add $1.25 for the first book, and $.25 for each additional book to cover postage and handling. Send check or money order only—no CODs) or charge my VISA, MASTERCARD or AMERICAN EXPRESS card.

Card number _____

Expiration date _____ Signature _____

Name _____

Address _____

City _____ State/Zip _____

Please allow six weeks for delivery. Prices subject to change without notice. Payment in U.S. funds only. New York residents add applicable sales tax.

TLP 12/88

Self-Help Guides
from St. Martin's Paperbacks

HOW TO SAVE YOUR TROUBLED MARRIAGE
Cristy Lane and Dr. Laura Ann Stevens
___ 91360-5 $3.50 U.S.   ___ 91361-3 $4.50 Can.

THE WAY UP FROM DOWN
Priscilla Slagle, M.D.
___ 91106-8 $4.50 U.S.   ___ 91107-6 $5.50 Can.

IN SEARCH OF MYSELF AND OTHER CHILDREN
Eda Le Shan
___ 91272-2 $3.50 U.S.   ___ 91273-0 $4.50 Can.

LOOK BEFORE YOU LOVE
Melissa Sands
___ 90672-2 $3.95 U.S.   ___ 90673-0 $4.95 Can.

SELF-ESTEEM
Mathew McKay and Patrick Fanning
___ 90443-6 $4.95 U.S.   ___ 90444-4 $5.95 Can.

Publishers Book and Audio Mailing Service
P.O. Box 120159, Staten Island, NY 10312-0004

Please send me the book(s) I have checked above. I am enclosing $_____ (please add $1.25 for the first book, and $.25 for each additional book to cover postage and handling. Send check or money order only—no CODs) or charge my VISA, MASTERCARD or AMERICAN EXPRESS card.

Card number _____

Expiration date _____ Signature_____

Name _____
Address _____
City _____ State/Zip _____

Please allow six weeks for delivery. Prices subject to change without notice. Payment in U.S. funds only. New York residents add applicable sales tax.

HELP 2/89